CONTACT DOUG AT

www.DougCrouse.com

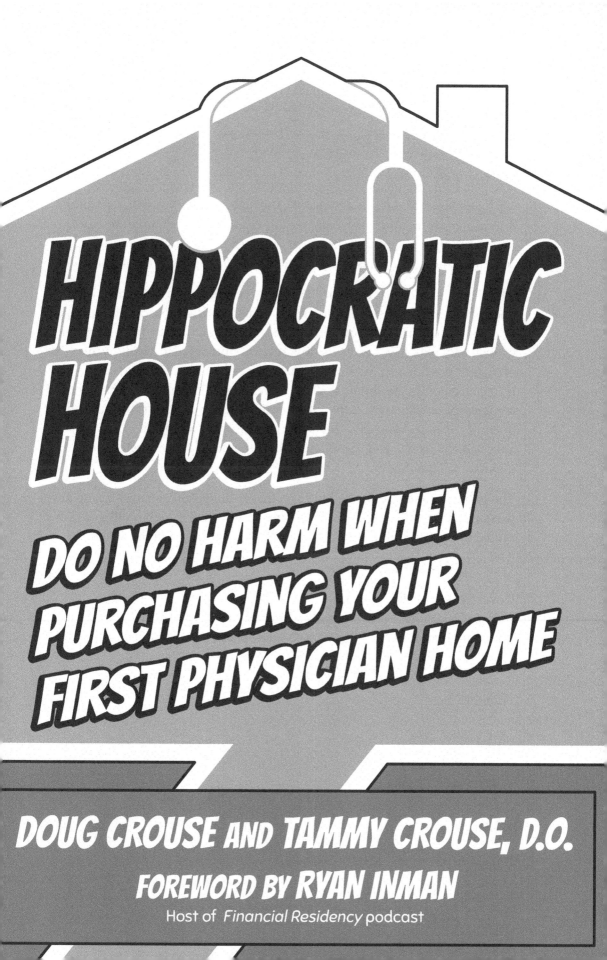

HIPPOCRATIC HOUSE

DO NO HARM WHEN PURCHASING YOUR FIRST PHYSICIAN HOME

DOUG CROUSE AND **TAMMY CROUSE, D.O.**

FOREWORD BY RYAN INMAN

Host of *Financial Residency* podcast

The Hippocratic House
Do No Harm When Purchasing Your First Physician Home
By Doug Crouse with Tammy Crouse, D.O.
Doug Crouse © 2021

Print ISBN: 978-1-61206-240-2

Cover Design by: Jon Herzog
Interior Design by: Rachel Langaker
Editorial Team: Jennifer Regner and Megan Terry

For more information, visit DougCrouse.com

Published by

ALOHA
PUBLISHING

AlohaPublishing.com

Printed in the United States of America

This book is dedicated to all the hard-working physicians who work tirelessly to keep us healthy and safe through COVID-19 and beyond. Thank you to each and every one of you for all you do. I have a front-row seat on what a day in the life of a doctor is like, being married to a physician myself. I am sure you don't hear this nearly enough. THANK YOU!

CONTENTS

FOREWORD

There is an art to buying your home as a physician family. It involves a lot of moving pieces, especially when it's your first home. However, armed with the right information, you'll be prepared to navigate the process smoothly.

Doug and Dr. Tammy Crouse are a physician family with the same concerns many physicians have about the homebuying process. They have walked the same road and faced the same challenges. Doug works full time in the mortgage industry helping physicians and their families understand the best lifestyle options, financing choices, and lending options for a home purchase. Whether you're about to purchase your first home or your second or third, their insights will help you become more comfortable with every step of the process. You'll learn everything you need to know, from prequalifying for a loan and finding the right lender to shopping for a house, negotiating, and closing. They'll help you understand how much house you can afford and whether now is the right time to buy.

Being married to a physician, I know the struggles you'll endure at different stages of your life. That's why it's become my mission to help doctors feel less overwhelmed with their money, so they can focus on the things that really matter. I want to ensure that you have a good experience buying your first home and make the right decisions for your family and your future.

My wife, Taylor, who is a pediatric pulmonologist, and I have seen families love their first home and others regret their decision. The difference? The latter didn't take just a little bit more time to intentionally plan for their homebuying opportunity. You can throw caution to the wind, buy the wrong house, and loathingly pay for it every month. Or, you can take a small amount of time to understand the real estate industry in order to make the best decisions about this important purchase.

Every physician family is unique in their needs and desires. That's why I encourage you to carefully consider your goals as you go into purchasing a home. Take a moment as you read this book to answer this question: What does your ideal life look like? Once you've envisioned that, it's easier to see where homeownership fits into that picture, and it gives you something to check your decisions against. Does buying a bigger home fit into the plan to create your ideal life? If you're someone who wants to spend more of your money on traveling, it may be beneficial to choose a smaller home—after all, you don't plan to spend as much time there anyway. But if your dream is to have a large yard where you can frequently host parties, maybe it's worth spending the extra money to have a larger chunk of land. The point of having a financial plan is to help you achieve your goals. You can spend your money however you want, but when you spend it in one place, it's no longer available to spend somewhere else. Know your priorities before you look for a house.

No part of the real estate market is one-size-fits-all. As a physician, you have unique opportunities for purchasing a home, including specialized loan products directed at doctors with extremely beneficial terms. As a mortgage expert, Doug Crouse will help you learn how to take advantage of these opportunities and understand the specifics of the process that apply to your situation.

Finding the right house in the right location with the best terms will bring you peace every day when you pull into your driveway. Moving out of a rental and into your first home, where you're building equity rather than spending money on rent, can be an incredible experience. And while the purchase process may seem intimidating at first, choosing a new home can be an adventure—a potentially stressful adventure, to be sure. With the right information, however, buying a home can and will go smoothly for you.

Ryan Inman
Host of *Financial Residency* podcast
Author of *Financial Residency: Create Your Financial Plan Without the Long Hours or Sleepless Nights*

INTRODUCTION

Buying your first house is a big deal. It's a lot of money on the line when you don't know how the process works. And like many physicians, if you are doing this as you transition from residency to your first job—that's another huge step in your life. You're trying to pack up, move, figure out licensing and privileges with your new position, and it's rush, rush, rush—you don't have time for anything, much less researching how to find a real estate agent and understand your financing options. I know this because I've been through it with my physician wife, Tammy. We wrote this book to make the crazy experience of buying your first home a little smoother for you.

We want to show you the process from beginning to end because there's a lot of misconceptions about your financing options, especially around physician loans. Plus, there's so many decisions to make. How do you pick the right real estate agent? How do you determine what price range you should be in? The typical "doctor house" will be well above $500,000 in many areas of the country. That's a lot, especially for your first time.

You'll work with two important people who will help you with the home-buying process: a lender and a real estate agent. We want you to *know* when you're talking with the right lender and the right real estate agent, and know what you're looking for instead of expecting them to educate you.

We want you to understand the process so you can make good decisions, ask the right questions, and keep your paperwork organized and somewhere that's accessible—instead of packed in a box in the back of a moving truck where you can't get it.

I know the mortgage industry well—I closed on 40 mortgages during the month I started writing this book, and I specialize in physician mortgages. Before I moved into financing, I sold houses for years and I've closed on 125 houses as a real estate agent, in addition to 20 years doing mortgage financing. I don't sell houses anymore, but I am in contact with many agents as a part of my day-to-day business.

What's the First Step?

First, you need to evaluate if this is the right time for you to buy. There's no harm or shame in renting for a while, especially if you're moving to a new city. It's great to get to know the area and figure out what parts of town you like and know for sure you want to stay there.

Once you've decided it's the right time, figure out how much you can afford and how much you're comfortable with spending. Only you know where your comfort level is with a monthly payment.

Understand that you can't necessarily equate the monthly payment you want with the principal and interest total you get from a mortgage calculator. Local taxes, homeowners insurance, and HOA dues can add significantly to that monthly payment. So you need to get a handle on that for your area too.

Once you know what kind of monthly payment you are comfortable with, it's time to find out how much house that payment can buy. To do that, you need to talk to a lender.

Connect With a Lender Before You Go Shopping

The lender should be your first stop before you go house hunting. Local taxes vary a lot and lenders will know how much cost the taxes will add. It's disappointing to fall in love with a $700,000 house and then find out you can only afford $500,000. It's better to know where to start up front and avoid the heartache.

So shop for a lender first, before you shop for a house. And approach it the same way—contact at least two to three lenders and get numbers from all of them, so you know what their fees are. All lenders are not the same and their fees can vary significantly. You can waste money in multiple places during a real estate transaction, and origination fees and the loan interest rates are two of the important ones. We'll show you what to look for and what's reasonable.

Also understand that the best lender for you may not be local. Your lender doesn't have to be within your state. I work in quite a few states and never meet most of my clients face to face.

The financing options can be one of the most confusing as well as important parts of the homebuying process. We'll explain what's different about a physician mortgage compared to conventional mortgage loans, so you know what to look for and can find a lender who specializes in that kind of loan.

STEP BY STEP: THE HOMEBUYING PROCESS

1. **Decide if now is a good time for you to buy.**

Consider your finances, career, family, and plans.

2. **Determine how much you can afford in a mortgage payment.**

Evaluate your current income, debt, and monthly expenses before taking the leap of buying a house. Make the decision for yourself and don't rely on what a bank or real estate agent tells you. Get all the papers together you'll need for the loan application and keep them accessible if you are moving.

3. **Connect with a lender, find out how much house you can afford, and get preapproved.**

All lenders are not the same. Shop for a lender and find one who can advise you on the best mortgage loan for you. Go through the preapproval process so you know how much house your monthly payment will buy. A lender can also connect you with excellent real estate agents, or an agent can help you get connected with a lender, if you find an agent first.

4. **Shop for a real estate agent and start looking at houses.**

Find an agent who's experienced and knowledgeable in the kinds of houses and neighborhoods you want to live in. They should look out for your best interests and help you find the house that fits your life. They should help you understand current market conditions and how to evaluate properties. Consider school districts, neighborhoods, and surrounding community amenities as you shop.

5. **Find the house you want and make an offer.**

Both your agent and your lender will be involved at this stage to put together an offer and the contract, advise you on contingencies for both finances and the real estate property, and assist with the negotiations.

6. **Sign the contract and start moving forward to the closing.**

Try to do home inspections ahead of the appraisal. Move forward on clearing all the contingencies, including sale of a current house if the new one is not your first. Lock in your interest rate if you haven't already. Provide updated paperwork to your lender as needed.

7. **Close on the property and move in.**

Warm up your signing hand and get the cash you'll need at closing ready. Coordinate moving companies, utility billing information and dates for transfer in your new house, and any repair, renovation, or updates to your new house. Move in!

Grand Rounds by Dr. Tammy

Make your first home purchase a Hippocratic house. Do no harm to your finances, your peace of mind, or your family's lifestyle with the choices you make. How can you do this? Knowledge. Real estate transactions and getting a mortgage are black boxes for many people, even after they've been through it once or twice. With this book, you can walk into the homebuying process with your eyes open and a good grasp on the terms and what's important for you to know. You'll know the right questions to ask and how to prepare.

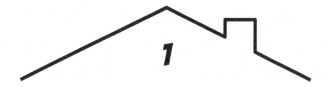

IS NOW THE RIGHT TIME FOR YOU TO BUY A HOUSE?

Why Should You Consider Buying a House?

For physicians, it's easy to think you can't possibly own a house when you have a lot of debt. But buying a house is a realistic option for many physicians, and your student loan balance isn't at the top of the list of important factors to consider. Debt can overshadow many other future plans, like starting a family or simply taking a vacation, but homeownership has benefits—it can improve your quality of life as well as your financial portfolio. If you do it right, you can handle both paying off your debts and learning the ropes of homeownership and still come out ahead in your finances.

A House Is an Investment

Owning a house gives you an opportunity to build some equity in the property as you make mortgage payments, while paying rent is simply spending money. By purchasing a house, you can get some return on the investment you make *and* a place to live.

If you consider that you'll always be making a monthly housing payment, whether it's rent into someone else's pocket or a mortgage payment on your own house, then your investment in a house is simply your down payment. That means the leveraging opportunity for your primary residence investment is huge.

Let's say you bought a $1,000,000 house and you put $50,000 down. You put 5% down and then the market goes up 5% a year. In two years, you'd have made a 200% return on your money (using simple interest, you made $50,000 per year for a new house value of $1,100,000 with $150,000 equity—not including the equity built up from the payments). The rest of it was the bank's money that you leveraged. So real estate, if done properly, absolutely beats the stock market as an investment, hand over fist.

Physicians often have a lot of student loan debt, but they also have financing options others don't. It's well known in the real estate industry that doctors are much less likely to default on a mortgage loan than the general public. You can benefit from the special loan products lenders offer to physicians.

The Timing Needs to Be Right

What you need to consider before you buy, that's more important than your student loan balance, is this: Are you planning to stay in the area for a while?

Buying a house costs a lot of money, before you've even moved in or made the first monthly payment. If you only live in the house for a year and then have to sell, you're probably better off renting. If you add the closing costs and fees you paid at closing to the monthly mortgage payment, and you sell in just a year or two, you may be paying more than the going rate for rent—plus there's a risk you'll lose money on the sale.

So unless you plan to keep the house and rent it after you move out, don't buy if you plan to move within a short period of time—or if you're uncertain about where you'll be in a few months.

Think Twice If You're a Resident

If you are a resident, buying a home should be considered carefully. The right choice for many residents is to rent. Your workload as a resident is overwhelming without any other responsibilities. A house requires upkeep, and the home-buying process itself takes time and energy. Also, because residents aren't yet making an attending salary, your financing options are more limited. While lenders specializing in physician loans do offer financing to residents, the best physician mortgage loan terms are usually reserved for attendings.

The temporary nature of resident positions is another good reason to put off buying a home until you're in a more stable situation. Similarly, if you're in your first job out of residency, you may also be better off renting for a year or more to find out if it's the right job and the right location for you.

Top Three Considerations to Help You Decide

Whether or not now is the right time to buy a house depends on several factors, including your student loan debt and your salary, but you need to consider your life circumstances along with your finances. There is no single right answer.

Your decision-making process should include these primary considerations:

1. Timing: Where are you in your career?
2. Finances: What can you afford and are you ready for the added expenses?
3. Renting versus buying: Which works better for you?

Timing

Just as in other big decisions, where you are in your career is a primary decision-making consideration for physicians who are thinking of buying a house. If you are still in med school, you likely can't qualify for a mortgage, and buying a house wouldn't be a good idea for many reasons. As a resident, your income has improved but the student loan debt can be a challenge to pay off; adding a mortgage payment may stretch your income too far. Add to that the crazy hours, and letting someone else fix the toilet can seem like a great idea.

While many physicians move for their first job out of residency and buy a house without considering renting for the first year or so, there's a chance you'll be changing jobs or locations a lot sooner than you think. If you are starting a new job, it's a good idea to evaluate the local job market for alternatives in case you don't like the position. That way, you may not have to move if you decide you want to change jobs.

A significant percentage of physicians find out they don't like their job after the first year or so, and many tend to change jobs every three to five years. They are sometimes forced to sell a house they just bought. This can have a big financial and personal impact on your life—extra expenses and extra stress.

Also, think about where you'd like to live long term. If you are a resident, think about how long your residency is, where the program is located, and what the job prospects as an attending in the area might be. If it's in an area where you'd like to stay, buying is a reasonable option. For example, if you are a resident with children and are living in your hometown, it could be more beneficial to buy a home rather than rent, depending on the market conditions in the area.

If you know for a fact that you *don't* want to live where you matched residency, you should carefully weigh your options before buying a house.

Another aspect to timing is the current state of the housing market where you want to buy. If your chosen area is a hot market, you may not get the value you desire from the purchase. You may have to offer more than the asking price to outcompete other buyers. Inventory may be limited and you may feel forced to buy a house that isn't really what you want. On the other hand, if the market is expected to continue to rise, you may decide to jump in rather than wait a year and discover that housing prices have increased by 10% and will cost you that much more. Researching market projections with the help of your lender or real estate agent can help you in this regard.

Finances

Your current financial status is another critical part of the homebuying decision. Where do you need to prioritize your money right now? If you have significant student loan debt, credit card debt, and no emergency fund, what do you need to have in place to feel more financially secure?

Evaluate Your Priorities

The biggest mistake many physicians make is buying more house than they need, or than they can afford at this point in their financial lives. If you still have significant debt from medical school or for any other reason, put the "doctor house" idea on hold. You may still be able to buy a house but consider it a starter home that you can live in comfortably while you pay off your other debts.

If you have a family to support, your priorities will be different than if you are single. Take the time to evaluate your financial situation, think about your financial goals, and make a plan for how to achieve your goals. Taking on a big house loan before you have a plan could stretch out your student loan payments for many years.

If you have no emergency fund and you are carrying a credit card balance, in addition to student loan debt, make a plan for creating a small emergency fund and contributing to it regularly—and get aggressive about paying off the credit cards. The house may need to wait until you're in a more secure financial position. See the Resources section at the end of this book for tools to help you evaluate your financial priorities.

When you buy a house, your monthly living expenses might increase. You should continue contributing regularly to your emergency fund to cover those increases and to build a bigger cushion.

If you've got room in the budget for your emergency fund contributions, student loan payments, and other life goals—in addition to the monthly payment and other expenses owning a house requires—you may be ready for homeownership.

Before you take on homeownership, have a good handle on your student loan debt. If you don't know exactly what your total debt is and what your repayment options are, get that information before going any further. You need to know how much of your monthly income will be tied up in loan repayments before you can figure out how big a mortgage payment you can afford. You can find tools for determining your student loan repayment options in the Resources section of this book.

Saving for a Down Payment Isn't Your First Priority

Many physicians think they need to save for a down payment, when they actually have other financial needs that should be addressed first. Once you put a down payment on a house, that money is tied up and can't be used elsewhere. Especially in uncertain times, it's best to put that money into an emergency fund, not the house. As a physician, you can find financing opportunities with competitive interest rates through physician mortgage loan financing that doesn't require a down payment.

The key is to understand your financial situation. Educate yourself because even if now isn't the right time, you'll know for sure when it is once you understand the whole process and what's required.

What's in Your Savings Account?

Buying a house costs money for the real estate transaction itself, called closing costs. So even if you decide to finance 100% and don't need money for the down payment, you will still have to pay the closing costs and expenses related to the transaction in cash at the closing. These expenses vary widely depending on local taxes, fees charged by the lender and the title company, current interest rates, and the house purchase price. Even for a $300,000 house, these fees can be in the neighborhood of $4,000 to $5,000, and the bigger the house, the more these will cost. If you don't have this plus some extra "just in case" set aside in your savings account, now isn't the time to buy.

Renting Versus Buying

The decision to rent or buy needs to take both timing and finances into account, plus your longer-term goals and your family situation and needs. There's much more to the decision whether to buy or rent than the size of the monthly payment and the house's investment potential. It also depends on the current housing market, where you are in your career and your life, and what is best for you and for others in your family.

If you know your current location isn't where you want to live long term, renting will simplify the move. However if you plan to keep the house and become a landlord after you move, buying a house while you're still in residency or during the first years of a new job can be a good plan—especially if you choose the house with renting it in mind, instead of looking for your "forever" home.

In fact, it's smart to look at any home purchase with an exit strategy in mind—either renting it or selling it—so you can easily do that when needed. Look at a home's desirability from a potential buyer's point of view, in addition to the features you want for yourself and your family. For many people, their "forever" home really means no more than 10 years and often it's less than that. Things can change unexpectedly, making everything look different.

You are probably already familiar with the ups and downs of renting, and it also helps to understand specific advantages and disadvantages to buying, so you can choose the option that fits you best—your personality, circumstances, and your long-term goals. Also see the list of advantages and disadvantages for both renting and buying near the end of this chapter.

A rent-or-buy calculator can help you determine whether renting or buying makes more financial sense for you. A link to one is included in the Resources section.

Advantages and Disadvantages to Homeownership

One of the biggest pluses to owning a home is the investment potential. You will build equity as you pay down the loan, and the property appreciation can help you build wealth over time. In addition to being a long-term investment, house ownership is also about creating stability, putting down roots, and building a life. If you have children, you may need the stability of homeownership for your family. Staying in the same neighborhood for your children's developing years can be a big part of providing them with the kind of childhood you want them to have.

The monthly mortgage payment also tends to be fairly stable. If you have a fixed-rate mortgage, your monthly principal and interest won't change over the life of the loan. Your property taxes might fluctuate a bit annually—and if property taxes go up, the value of your property is also going up, which is good. Even if you have an adjustable-rate mortgage, you will still know what to expect from your monthly payment, while rent could go up every year.

The interest you pay on your mortgage loan may be tax deductible. Tax laws change, so check with your accountant to make sure you are taking advantage of the available deductions. Another important advantage is that just like making regular student loan payments, owning a house builds your credit.

Many consider homeownership one of the keys to a better quality of life, especially if it provides you with the privacy, surroundings, and "room to breathe" that you desire. Because you own the property, you can upgrade or renovate your house and yard. The more important those intangible things are to you, the more willing you will be to take on the expenses and responsibilities that come with owning a home.

The disadvantages of buying a home are tied to the investment risk, the expenses, and the responsibilities of owning a home. Just like any investment, there is risk associated with buying a house. The housing market could crash and the value of your house could drop below the purchase price. If you financed 100% of your purchase price, you could be "underwater" on your home—meaning you owe more than it's worth. This isn't a catastrophe if you don't have to sell right now because you can ride it out until the market recovers. Having some equity in the house can protect you somewhat in that event.

If you need to move unexpectedly, you may not get the value of your closing costs back. So there's risk that you can lose money if you are forced to sell in a short time after buying. Also, mortgage payments are structured initially to put almost all of each payment toward interest and not your principal balance. This means you don't build much equity in the house in the first few years of mortgage payments—another reason why it can be detrimental to sell soon after the purchase.

Historically, real estate has proven to be one of the best risks a person can take in the long run. If you're betting on something by taking out loans, there are two bets statistically worth taking: medical school and a home loan.

In terms of expenses, closing costs are an expense you must pay to complete the real estate transaction to own a home. In addition, the down payment can be a large expense, but as a physician, you are generally eligible to finance up to 100% of the loan, unlike most people. This is a tremendous benefit because saving the traditional 20% of a house purchase price can take years. So this one doesn't apply to everyone.

Other expenses of homeownership include homeowners insurance and the cost of utilities, and you need to include them in calculating what you can afford to spend on a home. Electricity, natural gas, water, internet service, and possibly cable or phone bills all add to the monthly expenses. Electricity might be the biggest wild card, depending on local climate and rates. The hotter the summer, the more you will need to run your air conditioning. People with longer, colder winters will have higher heating bills.

The size of the house matters too. Heating and cooling a 1,000 square foot apartment or house could cost considerably less than it would for a 3,000 square foot house—although energy efficiency can make a big difference. When you are house shopping, ask your real estate agent for estimated utility costs from the previous owner.

Owning a home means being responsible for making sure it is maintained and operational. Maintenance and repairs can take significant time from your nights and weekends. You need to be willing to do this or hire someone else to do it. The heating and cooling system need maintenance and eventually repair or replacement. Windows, appliances, plumbing, gutters, paint, and other things will all need attention at some point. Mowing the lawn, pulling weeds, and trimming shrubs and trees will take time away from your rest and relaxation.

A new house will need less maintenance (at least initially) than one that's 40 years old, so keep that in mind when you're shopping too. If you know you will have many on-call days, don't buy a fixer-upper.

Summary: Upsides and Downsides to Buying

Here is a summary of the upsides and downsides to buying and owning a home.

Upsides to Buying a House

- Investment potential

- Stability

- Tax-deductible interest

- Credit-building potential

- Quality of life, including the freedom to change or renovate

Downsides to Buying a House

- Risk tied to the investment and housing market health

- Expenses including the down payment, closing costs, homeowners insurance, monthly utilities, and maintenance and repair

- Responsibility for keeping the property looking good and operational

Summary: Upsides and Downsides to Renting

People tend to think of the downsides to renting, but there are some upsides too—especially if flexibility is important to you.

Upsides to Renting

- No maintenance or repairs: Someone else fixes things when they break, and they pay for it too.

- For apartments and condos: No yardwork. This one may not apply if you rent a house.

- Flexibility: You have no long-term commitment, so job changes that require moving are easier and faster to handle.

- Value: Depending on the local housing market, you may be able to afford to rent in an area you couldn't afford to buy in.

- Lower costs: You may need to pay only a deposit and one or two months' rent before moving in. You need only renters insurance to cover your belongings, instead of homeowners insurance to cover the property and liability as well.

Downsides to Renting

- Noisy or transitional neighbors: Especially in an apartment or condo, your neighbors may be less considerate than you would like, making noise and other problems that add stress and distraction to your life.

- Restrictions on personalizing your space: If your surroundings are important to you, not being able to choose something as basic as the color of the walls without permission from a landlord can be frustrating.

- No control over rent increases: When the rent goes up, your only options are to pay it or move out.

- Lease agreement limitations: As a tenant, you are bound by the rules of the agreement. You can't make changes to a rented property without communicating with and obtaining consent from the owner.

- Rental liaison: You may have to deal with a property management company or rental agent, acting as a liaison between you and the owner. Approvals for repairs and other issues may take longer to resolve as a result.

- No investment potential: Your monthly payments don't go toward building equity when you rent. For many people, this makes renting a short-term proposition. From a personal wealth standpoint, you are likely better off buying if you will stay there for more than five years.

Know Your Credit Score

Your credit score represents a measure of risk to a lender. It is a number of 850 or less, calculated from the information in your credit report. The higher your score is, the less risk there will be to a lender—that is, the more likely you are to responsibly pay your debts.

If you have student loans and have been paying on them for a while, you've had opportunities to build a good score. If you are married, you should know your spouse's score too. You have the option of doing a joint application and may need to do that, depending on your circumstances. If your spouse's income is part of the qualification, then they need to be on it.

If your spouse's income is not needed but they have a better credit score than yours, you'll want to include them on the application. If their score is not as good as yours and their income is not needed, it's probably better to leave them off the application.

Before you go shopping for a lender to buy your first house, find out what your credit score is. If your score isn't great there may be things you can do to improve it, but none of those actions will make a difference in 30 days. You need a few months or a year to make changes that could improve your score.

If your score is less than 680, it may not be the right time to buy a house until you can improve it. Renting for another year or two while you fix some of those issues will save you significant money.

How to Find Your Credit Score

You can obtain a free credit *report* once a year through an FTC (Federal Trade Commission) endorsed website, but it will not include your credit *score*. Be aware that there are different algorithms used to calculate the actual score number and the results may vary somewhat from one source to the next. The number you obtain may not be exactly what the mortgage lender will see, but it will be close enough and will give you an idea of your status.

Obtaining your credit score is a different process from obtaining your report. If you have a credit monitoring service to protect you against identity theft, you can obtain a credit score through that service (if you don't have such a service, now may be a good time to get one). Credit card companies and banks may offer a free credit score as part of their services, and you can reach out to their customer service to request it.

What's High Enough?

Credit is a large part of the qualification process for a mortgage loan. A lender will look at both your credit score and your credit report. Your credit score can impact how much interest you are charged for a loan. The higher your credit score, the better your interest rate will be, plus other terms will be more advantageous too. A credit score of 760 or higher will get you the best interest rate possible. Someone with a lower score, indicating a greater risk of default, will pay a higher interest rate.

> A high credit score will give you a better interest rate.

Insurance companies and lenders of all types base the rates they charge you on your credit score as well, so the savings aren't just from mortgage loan financing. Every lender has their own criteria, but as a rule of thumb, many don't go below 700 for physician loans and some may require 720 or as high as 740. The lowest I've seen accepted is 680.

For other types of mortgage loans, the credit score requirements will be different and the acceptable range much wider, but your terms will reflect where your score falls.

Understanding Credit Reports and Credit Scores

Your credit *report* is a detailed history of current and past credit accounts and their current status. Three credit reporting agencies maintain a credit report on you, starting with when you first open a credit account.

Your credit *score* is built from your credit report. The lower the score, the more likely you are to miss payments or go into default.

There are three major credit reporting agencies:

- Equifax

- Experian

- Transunion

They gather information from anyone you've done business with. They find out if you've been on time, been late, or if you've ever defaulted on payments. Several categories of financial transactions are pulled together for your credit report and influence your credit score:

- Paying bills on time

- Credit history

- Credit types

- Debt-to-credit ratio (credit utilization)

See the Resources section for a website link for free credit reports.

Check Your Credit Report for Discrepancies

Obtaining a free credit report is relatively easy. See the Resources page for a link to the free report recommended by the U.S. FTC (Federal Trade Commission).

You should check your credit score and your report about once a year, whether you are thinking of making a major purchase or not.

With the increased incidence of identity theft, it's not uncommon to pay for a credit-monitoring service that keeps an eye on your credit report and will let you know of any changes or suspicious activity. When you review your report, look at every item to make sure you recognize it. Check the report from each of the three agencies. You may find a discrepancy on one and not the others.

It is quite common to find mistakes on a credit report. If you find an error, you can take action to have it corrected.

What to Do If You Find a Mistake in Your Credit Report

Write a letter to the credit bureau detailing why the reported information is wrong (or submit this information online). If your report has the same mistake from all three reporting agencies, you need to contact each one. You can find sample dispute letters online.

Provide a copy of any supporting documents (always keep your originals). It will take 30 days for the credit bureau to investigate and another five to send the results.

If something was corrected, you can ask the credit reporting agency to send an updated copy to anyone who received the erroneous report in the last six months, or to an employer who requested it within the past two years.

Building a Good Credit Score: Pay Your Bills on Time

The basis for good credit is punctual and consistent payment of debts. If you were late with a single payment at some point in your history, the damage is temporary. If you are consistently late or have missed multiple payments, your score will be affected. So if you've been making on-time student loan payments for four years in residency and haven't carried big credit card balances or missed a lot of payments, you should have a decent credit score.

Credit Inquiries

Anytime someone runs a credit inquiry, you will get a "hit" to your credit score, which will lower it. There's no way around it. A credit inquiry is related to your applying for credit: applying for a new credit card or financing for any purchase. How many points off your score that hit will cost depends on how many credit cards you have open and your credit profile.

However, this drop in your score is not permanent. You will likely get 50% of your points back at the end of 30 days, and in two months the points you lost will be back. This is why you don't want to make any changes or applications for any other kind of financing too close to your application for a mortgage loan.

How to Improve Your Credit Score

If your score isn't where you want it to be, here are some things you can do.

If your score is low because of late or missed payments, only time without another incident can fix that. Carrying a balance on your credit cards, especially if it is over 30% of the credit limit, will hurt your score and paying down that debt will improve it.

A medical collection will hurt your score. However, if it's two years old, paying it now will not help—it essentially takes something that was old and makes it current.

For many physicians, what hurts their credit is over-utilization of credit cards. Over-utilized credit means having a balance of more than 30% of your credit limit *on any one card*. The more often this happens, the more your score will drop. So if you have maxed out credit cards or anything over 50% of your credit limit, your score will definitely be hurt by that. Requesting a higher credit limit can help bring that percentage down and may be your only option if you can't afford to pay it off yet. A similar solution is opening a new line of credit and transferring some of the balance to it. Your score will take a temporary hit (a few months) from the act of opening a new credit card account.

What matters is the utilization percentage *per card*—not in total. So if you use one card all the time and have a balance well over 30% of your credit limit, and you have two other cards with no balance at all, your credit score will improve if you spread out the card usage so none of them go over 30%. Once you make that change, it will take time to reflect in your score. So none of these things will help you in a month.

Example: Oscar has five credit cards. Each credit card has a $30,000 limit. Oscar spends $2,000 on each card. That makes his utilization low for each card—less than 10%.

Here is another example: Oscar has 10 credit cards. On one card he put $5,000 (the card has a limit of $10,000). The utilization looks good on the other nine cards. The utilization looks bad on the card with $5,000.

Why does it look bad on the card with $5,000? The answer is because he has spent half the credit available to him. His utilization ratio is too high.

If you are a new attending physician with a solid credit history, you may also have a lower credit score because your student loans are maxed out due to the fact that you are in forbearance—you haven't started paying them. This is why your utilization may be high early in your career. (Lenders know this about physicians and will typically ignore the impact of student loans on your score—but your credit card balances still matter.)

To keep your revolving credit utilization below 30%, ask for a higher credit limit than you need and charge no more than 30% of each card's limit so you are not penalized.

Other things that will improve your score include minimizing missed payments, not carrying a balance on your credit cards (paying them off in full each month), and paying off other kinds of debt (student loans, vehicle loans, and any other kind of loan).

What builds a high credit rating is low debt utilization, no negative events, and a long history. A record of debts paid as agreed is also a big boost. You can improve your score by being added as an authorized user on someone else's account that has those things—say, a $40K credit limit card with no balance that's 10 years old. If your score is 640 due to some things out of your control in the past, in addition to not repeating those things and keeping your credit utilization under 30% on each credit card, you can improve your score by getting added as an authorized user to someone's account with low debt utilization and a long history. Again, you won't see the results of this overnight.

Having more credit cards may or may not improve your credit score. It all depends on how you handle the accounts. How many credit cards is ideal? There isn't a hard-and-fast rule. You don't want so many that keeping track of your accounts becomes a nightmare. You probably want to have at least three credit cards—a primary, a backup (in case the primary is hacked), and a third option.

If you do have several credit cards and decide you want to cut down on the number, don't get rid of any that have a long history, if you have a choice. That history will benefit you when it's time to improve your credit score. And again, don't decide to close any immediately before applying for a mortgage loan or financing for any big purchase.

You can help your children build credit before they need it by adding them as an authorized user on one of your credit card accounts. By the time they have a credit card of their own, they will have a long history of good credit utilization, even if they never used that card.

Credit scores are also based on how many accounts you have. If you have a history of paying credit over several accounts, it will improve your credit score.

Other Aspects of Credit

Mortgage loan underwriters look for the same categories that influence your credit score (repayment history), but they also look at your employment history, income, and debts. They will look through your finances with a fine-toothed comb: savings, checking accounts, and other types of financial accounts. They will likely confirm your employment at least once. Lastly, they look at your debt-to-income ratio.

Underwriters want to know if you pay your bills on time, stay steadily employed, have assets (cash) in backup for worst-case situations or for a down payment, and don't carry too much debt. These things all indicate that your risk of default is low.

Notes on Damage Control

If your credit score is low because of things in your past that you can't change—such as making a car payment late or you've had a medical collection—time and no repeats of those events are the only things that will help. And concerning paying off a collection to help your score, about half the time paying an old medical collection will be worse than not paying it because something that was two years old has now been made current.

HIPPOCRATIC HOUSE CHECKLIST

Improving Your Credit Score for Mortgage Loan Underwriting

Your lender wants to know what kind of risk they are taking when they offer you a mortgage loan. A mortgage underwriter is the person who determines the risk that you would default on a loan.

If you are married, include your spouse on the loan application if you need their income or they have a better credit score than yours. If their score is worse than yours and you can meet the income requirements without them, it's best not to include them.

Your credit score will save or cost you money, depending on where it falls, so it's worth taking the time to improve it. If you have a few months' time before you will apply for a mortgage, try some of these steps to improve your score:

- ❑ Spread out your spending across several cards instead of putting it all on one card, to keep your utilization below 30% per card.

- ❑ Another way to improve (lower) credit utilization is to request an increased credit limit on the card(s) you use the most.

- ❑ Opening another credit line can improve your credit utilization, however your score will take a temporary hit for opening another account. So don't do that too close to when you want to apply.

- ❑ If the non-wage-earning spouse has a better credit score, include them on the application.

- ❑ If your spouse's score is higher, adding yourself as an approved user onto their card account can improve yours—if that account has a long credit history and low utilization.

- ❑ Pay off debt.

- ❑ Pay bills on time. Automate payments to make this easy.

- ❑ Check your credit report for errors.

HIPPOCRATIC HOUSE CHECKLIST

Are You Ready to Buy a House?

Here is a checklist to help you determine if you are ready to buy a house. The unexpected can happen to anyone, but being able to check off these things will help you know you are prepared and ready to take on homeownership.

- ❑ Stability: You and/or your family need or want the stability and comfort of a house, yard, and neighborhood.

- ❑ Timing: You are planning to stay in the area for the foreseeable future (at least a few years), in terms of your career and family/life goals.

- ❑ Workload: You are willing and able to spend time in the evenings and on weekends to keep your place looking good and maintained properly, or are prepared to hire these things out. You have time for the homebuying process.

- ❑ Financial goals: You know what your financial goals and priorities are, and homeownership is one of your priorities.

- ❑ Assets and income: You have enough money on hand to cover the closing costs required up front to purchase a house. Your budget can handle not only any student loan payments you need to make and the monthly mortgage payment, but also the utilities, insurance, and maintenance and repair expenses that go along with homeownership.

- ❑ Emergency Fund: You have a minimum of two to three months' worth of living expenses saved and readily accessible and have included continuing contributions in your budget projections for homeownership.

- ❑ Debt: You have a plan for repaying your student loans. You don't have a lot of consumer debt such as credit card balances or vehicle loans, and you've prioritized paying off any that you have in a reasonable amount of time.

❑ Credit score: Your score is 700 or more, allowing you access to great terms on physician loans or other types of financing.

You don't have to have all the answers right now. The next few sections will help you fill in the gaps and even if now isn't the right time, you'll be educated on the process and will know when it is the right time as a result.

Grand Rounds by Dr. Tammy

My motto at work is *"just because you can, doesn't mean you should."* I think this applies to home purchases as well. Up to 70% of physicians leave their first job within two years. Before you buy that expensive "forever" home, be sure you love your job and find the right neighborhood for you and your situation. Don't get locked into a job because you can't afford to leave your house.

Chapter 1 Takeaways

 Buying a home and taking on mortgage debt can be a sound real estate investment strategy, even if you have substantial student debt. Just make sure you can afford both the loan payments and the mortgage payment without making yourself house poor.

 Think carefully about buying a house when you are a resident. For many residents, renting lets you enjoy your time off without having to spend time making repairs, and gives you the flexibility to pick up and move whenever you like.

If you are an early-career physician, buying a house may complicate things for you, especially if you decide you don't like the job and need to move.

If you have significant consumer debt (credit cards, vehicle loans) and no emergency fund, you may be far better off waiting until you eliminate that debt and have at least a month or two of expenses stashed away in an emergency fund before you start house shopping.

Your credit report and your credit score are two different things, and you need to look at both. Getting your credit report is easy, and getting your credit score is getting easier. Knowing your credit score is a good thing to do before you make the decision to buy a house because if your score isn't great, there are things you can do to improve it, given a few months' time.

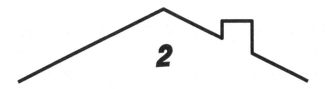

HOW MUCH HOUSE CAN YOU AFFORD?

Before you start shopping for a lender, a real estate agent, or a house, you need to determine the monthly house payment you'll be comfortable with. Evaluate your financial situation and your goals and decide this for yourself.

A lender or agent will often tell you what the maximum amount you can borrow is. If you go with that number, I guarantee you'll be house poor. Using their criteria, you'll be able to buy much more than you're comfortable with.

There's nothing wrong with buying a house commensurate with your income—just don't overdo it. Buying too much house is one of the most common mistakes physicians make. There's no reason to buy a house that's so expensive you end up living paycheck to paycheck on a physician's income.

Student loan debt can be a "gotcha" because lenders may overlook that debt when they estimate what you can borrow. Keep your student loan payments in mind, even if the lender is willing to overlook it. There's a big difference in available budget between a physician with no student loan debt and one that's sitting on $750,000 in debt.

Where you choose to live makes a huge difference in affordability, and you may not be able to afford the big "doctor's house" in some metropolitan areas. Housing prices relative to physician incomes can vary widely. In Los Angeles, $800,000 might buy a starter home while in Oklahoma, that's a mansion. When you choose to live on the East or West Coast on a doctor income, you might be an average income in certain zip codes. Physicians in LA are usually poorly paid because they live in a great climate, whereas a doctor in Oklahoma makes an income in the top 0.1%.

Another "gotcha" can be homeowners association fees. For any neighborhood you are considering, ask your agent to provide the HOA fee amounts for that area. Depending on local cost of living and amenities offered, these can range from a few hundred dollars per year to $1,200 per month or more. Condominiums tend to have high fees.

The key is to figure out for yourself what monthly payment you're comfortable committing to, figure out how much house that can buy, and shop in your price range. That way you won't go looking at houses you can't afford and feel disappointed when you realize you can't have it.

Good Debt Versus Bad Debt

Mortgage debt is considered by many to be good debt, or maybe not even considered to be debt at all. It's necessary debt for most because it's one of the biggest purchases you'll ever make. Medical school is also expensive, and can cost $50,000 or more per year. By the end of your training, you may have debt the size of a second mortgage, even before you buy a house.

You can think of your student loan debt as an investment in your earning potential. That's because your medical degree will earn you far more than the student loans are worth over the course of your working life.

While paying monthly rent gives you a place to live, buying a house not only gives you a place to live but an opportunity to build equity, month by month, in a real estate asset that can appreciate over time. It's an investment.

Good debt allows you to own something that appreciates in value and can give you a return on your investment. Both medical school loans and a mortgage to buy a house are good debts—the return on your investment could potentially be greater than what you contributed. As you pay them off, you also can build up your credit rating while gaining something of value.

An example of bad debt is a vehicle loan. While a vehicle is an asset, it starts losing value the day you drive it off the lot. It is not an investment and you want to minimize borrowing money to buy it as much as possible, and pay off the resulting debt as soon as possible.

Bad debt is debt used to buy something that won't appreciate over time to give you any kind of return. So a car loan, while it may be necessary, is bad debt and should be minimized as much as possible—and paid off as soon as possible.

Bad debt is also when you buy things you can't afford today and plan to pay off tomorrow. Running up charges on your credit cards is bad debt, and because the interest is typically much higher than either mortgages or vehicle loans, it should be avoided at all costs.

Many physicians feel that with student loans hanging over their heads, taking on another large loan to buy a house might not be the best idea. But mortgage debt can be part of a sound financial life plan—if you don't overspend on your house and jeopardize other categories in your budget. And as long as you don't go for too big a house, you can make choices so you can manage both your student loan payments and the mortgage payment with room to spare.

A Mortgage Is Still Debt

Some people don't actually think of mortgage debt as "real" debt, but it is—it is still a liability. It costs you something as long as you carry it. Just because you financed your house purchase with a 30-year loan doesn't mean you should take 30 years to pay it off. In fact, ideally you would make a plan from the beginning to pay it off much sooner.

If you have room in your budget, consider a 15-year mortgage. Shorter loans will have a higher monthly payment and a lower interest rate, and you will pay much less in interest over the life of the loan. If the payments are too high on the 15-year loan, another approach is to go for the 30-year loan but budget extra payments into your plan so you can pay off the loan in less time.

The benefits of owning your home free and clear cannot be underestimated. If you go into the purchase with that in mind, you can set up your best scenario to make it happen.

How Much Is Too Much House?

What's too much house depends on you and your family's needs and budget. A big mortgage can limit your options, if you discover you want to go to part time, retire early, or switch careers to something a little less lucrative but more satisfying. You have to determine what you can afford for yourself. Don't accept what anyone else tells you, including lenders and real estate agents.

You also have to be happy with how much money is left over each month after the bills, retirement, emergencies, and life plans have been covered. How important the house is to you is also part of the equation—your priorities.

To avoid buying too much house, educate yourself about the true cost of homeownership. The cost of owning a home is more than the monthly mortgage payment, so you need to be prepared for the all the ways a home costs you money. Even if you finance 100% of the purchase price (no down payment), you still have to have cash for the closing.

Here are the big categories of expenses you will take on to finance the house and complete the real estate transaction:

- Monthly mortgage payment: Principal and interest **plus** homeowners insurance and property taxes are typically included in the monthly payment. **You'll pay this for the life of the mortgage loan.**

- Closing costs: These are the combined fees from everyone who's involved in your house purchasing process. Closing costs depend on the purchase price of your house and the fees charged by the lender and real estate agents, along with others who provide services to complete the transaction. This is the cost of the homebuying transaction and must be paid at closing. More on this later.

- Down payment: This doesn't apply to everyone, but you should understand your options. If it's part of your deal, you must pay this with cash at closing. It can be up to 20% of the house purchase price or it can be zero, depending on your circumstances and the financing you set up with your lender.

Here's a list of additional ways you'll spend money as a homeowner, some of them soon after you move in:

- Furniture and household items: Moving from an apartment to a house may require a lot more furniture. Window coverings can be a significant expense category too.

- Landscaping: Fencing and new trees and shrubs plus a lawnmower, leaf blower, and weed trimmer are some of the things you may need to spend on.

- Repairs and maintenance: Estimate 1-3% of the purchase price of the house every year for typical upkeep.

- Utilities: Heating, cooling, internet, TV, water/sewer and trash service all must be paid monthly. The bigger the house, the bigger the heating and cooling bills will be, and these can be significant in very hot or cold climates. Utility rates also vary tremendously in different regions.

- Homeowners association (HOA) fees: Many subdivisions have a homeowner's association with associated fees to cover common area landscaping, insurance, and neighborhood amenities. These vary from a few hundred dollars a year to a large part of your monthly payment in high cost of living areas.

The cost of moving isn't included here because hopefully that will be paid by your employer—but if you intend to go into private practice, you may need to add that one to the list too.

How to Determine What You Can Afford

If you don't already have a monthly budget, take a moment to list your monthly income and expenses. Don't forget to save for retirement and include some money to do things you enjoy. Here's some of the information you'll need to make a decision on the size of mortgage payment you can live with:

1. **Money in:** Determine your take-home monthly income.

2. **Money out:** Make sure your budget projections include these things:

   a. The mortgage payment itself (an estimate—start with at least whatever you're paying now for rent)

   b. A monthly utilities estimate

c. An estimate on maintenance and repair costs (for instance, 1% of the loan amount)

d. Bills such as student loans and other loans

e. Contributions toward other life goals

f. Contributions to your emergency fund

g. Extra payments toward the mortgage principal (if it's your goal to pay it off early)

h. Living expenses: food, clothing, insurance, entertainment, etc.

If you have already determined your living expenses and have a plan for handling your student loan debt, you are ahead of the game. If you haven't done this yet, take the time to do it now, so you clearly understand what kind of mortgage payment you can afford.

The "gotcha" for physicians is the student loan debt some lenders will ignore. Lenders specializing in physician loans will often ignore your student loan debt when they calculate what you qualify for, so you have to determine for yourself what you're comfortable spending each month. Even if your loans are in deferment, do an analysis as if you were paying them to make sure you aren't stretching yourself too far.

The longer you stretch out your student loan payments, the more it will cost you, even if you have are in a PSLF (public service loan forgiveness) program. You still need to make the minimum 120 payments.

Once you are comfortable with your financial situation, you can make a good decision about how much of your monthly income you can commit to a mortgage payment.

Calculate a Mortgage Payment You Can Afford

What follows is a simple calculation to help you see the big picture on your finances and how a mortgage can fit in. Use this as a guideline.

Follow these steps to determine how much you can afford to spend on a house.

1. **Consider how much you're bringing in.**
   Add up all of your take-home monthly pay from all of your income sources. As an example, let's say your monthly take-home pay is $12,000.

   Take-home pay: _____

2. **Multiply your take-home pay by 25%.**
   Multiply your take-home pay by 25% (0.25) to get the maximum amount you can afford to spend monthly on your home. (This is not just your maximum mortgage payment. It is the maximum amount you can pay toward your mortgage payment plus all of the other expenses. Those expenses would include principal, interest, taxes, insurance, HOA dues, maintenance and repairs, and utilities. See step 3.)

   For example, $12,000 x 25% = $3,000.

   Take-home pay x 25% = _____

3. **Determine the extra expenses.**
   In the next step, we will determine principal, interest, taxes, and insurance (PITI). But before we get there, you need to determine what all your extra expenses are. Add up your HOA dues, any special assessments (such as additional property tax), and budget for deferred maintenance and repairs.

   With our example, we will use $500 a month as the total cost for these extra expenses.

   Extra expenses:

   _____   _____

   _____   _____

   Total = _____

4. **Use the mortgage calculator to determine your maximum mortgage payment.**

Now that we have determined the maximum amount you can afford to allocate in your budget to a home purchase (step 2), subtract the additional expenses from that number (as calculated in step 3) to determine the maximum mortgage payment you can afford each month. You can find a mortgage calculator in the Resources section of this book.

Here is an example to see how to work through it:

- $450,000 purchase price and loan amount at 3.75%

- $4,500 property tax (1% of purchase price), 0% down payment

- $600-per-year homeowners insurance

This will bring your monthly mortgage amount to $2,500—an amount you can realistically afford.

You can download this mortgage calculation as a PDF at DougCrouse.com

Translating the Mortgage Payment Into a House Purchase Price

So how much house will that buy? You'll need to talk to a lender and also know the cost of HOA dues for the subdivision you want to buy in to figure out what your purchase price can be, but here's an example of how it works.

If your take-home pay is $12,000 a month, that means the maximum amount you should allocate for a house is $3,000 a month (as calculated in step 2). If you have an additional $500 a month of extra expenses (as calculated in step 3), then you can afford a $450,000 house as shown above.

If you want to purchase a house that is more expensive, you will need to have a down payment to keep the monthly payment the same. For example, if the house is $500,000 and you keep everything else the same, you will need a $50,000 down payment.

A mortgage payment is made up of multiple parts—principal and interest, and one twelfth of property taxes, homeowners insurance, and sometimes the homeowners association dues. The current interest rate is also a big variable and the higher the interest rate, the less house you can afford.

How much taxes and insurance cost will vary by state, but as a rough estimate, a $4,500 payment might equate to a $750,000 house in an intermediate cost of living area. Your lender can help you with estimates on taxes and homeowners insurance and can give you interest rate ranges. In Texas, a third of the house payment might go toward taxes and insurance, while in other states, they might amount to 15% of the payment.

Another possible "gotcha" is the homeowners association fees; for some high cost of living areas like Hawaii, they can be more than $1,000 per month.

As you shop for lenders, tell them what monthly payment you'd like to have and ask them for a house price range you can use as you shop.

How Lenders Determine What You Can Afford

Lenders calculate the maximum amount they are willing to lend you based on the level of risk they take with you as a borrower. They will offer you an amount that is mathematically and statistically sound. It has nothing to do with what's reasonable or comfortable for you. You can always borrow less than the lender is willing to lend.

An industry standard approach is to start with 45% of your gross income and subtract out all *credit reportable debts* plus any child support or alimony.

As an example, for a $20,000 per month income, a physician could afford to spend $9,000 as a baseline. If they've got $400,000 in student loans, the monthly payment on those can be estimated at 1% of the balance, so that's a $4,000 payment. Now they can afford $5,000 for the house. Then subtract car loans and credit card minimum payments, and let's say those total another $500. So they can afford $4,500 and that's the maximum payment.

This is where the local housing market, current interest rates, and local taxes and fees must be taken into account. In a lower cost of living area with interest rates in the 3% range, they can probably afford a $750,000 house.

If this physician had no student loans, they could potentially afford nearly twice that much (an $8,500 payment), if having a big house is one of their life goals.

Don't Use the Number the Bank Gives You

It's important for you to know what you are comfortable committing to every month, before a lender gives you their number.

> It's almost certain that if you go with what the lender says you can afford, you'll be house poor.

Don't do it!

House poor means realizing at age 50 that you can't retire until age 65 because too much of your income went to the house instead of your retirement. It can also mean many other missed opportunities because your money is committed to the big house. Don't limit your career choices by tying yourself to a large mortgage payment. That payment can prevent you from changing careers to escape burnout, going to part-time work if you decide you want to, or retiring early.

Even if a big house is one of your life goals, wait until you're financially ready for a large mortgage. That means no student loan debt, a significant emergency fund stashed away, and a stable job, among other things.

When you first interview lenders, have an informal discussion about how much they think you can afford. This is not the preapproval process, which looks in depth at your financial liabilities and assets, but a higher-level discussion about what they think you can handle. The answers they provide can help you understand whether they are looking out for your interests or not, and help you determine if they are the right lender for you.

The two most important things to remember when starting the house-buying process are these:

1. Don't buy too much house.
2. Make sure you understand your debt.

Do You Need a Down Payment?

The short answer is no, probably not. If you are out of residency and have a decent credit rating, you can likely qualify for a physician mortgage with competitive terms—for up to 100% of the purchase amount. This is almost always the best way for physicians to finance with no down payment.

If you can put 20% down on a house purchase, you will have the best financing options available, hands down. You won't have to worry about the extra expense of private mortgage insurance (PMI), no matter what kind of loan you use, and you'll have that equity in the house from the day they hand you the keys.

However, many physicians don't have much in savings and there are often good reasons why you shouldn't wait to buy a house until you can save that money. If you want to buy a $500,000 house but have to wait three or four years to save up the $100,000 down payment, in many markets the house value will have increased so it will cost more. In an appreciating market, that could be 10-20% in appreciation. If you had bought the house right away with 0% down instead, that appreciation would contribute to your equity, along with the payments made during that time. Plus, it may be a better use of that money to pay down existing debt (with an interest rate higher than the rate of return you'll get on your house investment) or contribute to an emergency fund.

Having some equity in your house is a good thing, but if you invest that money elsewhere, it won't be tied up in a house and the risks that come with it. So if you need to sell your house and want to have 10% equity, put that 10% in a more accessible place rather than tied up in your house.

For most physicians, it doesn't make sense to postpone buying to save for a down payment, because you won't make any impact on the mortgage except a slightly lower monthly payment. For example, if you put $100,000 down on a house, that's going to save you $450 on your mortgage payment each month. But if you put $100,000 into paying off two cars, that might free up $1,500 in monthly payments.

Closing Costs

Buying a house costs money beyond what you pay every month on the mortgage. The real estate transaction itself costs money and the entire housing industry makes their money this way: lenders, real estate agents, title companies, house inspectors, and the list goes on. This is why a house is considered a long-term investment and why you may have heard that if you sell a house in less than five years after purchase you may lose money on the deal.

Even if you finance 100% of the purchase price, you still need to have money in your pocket to buy a house. You will pay closing costs and related expenses for the real estate transaction, and you must have this in cash. Closing costs are difficult to estimate because they depend heavily on local taxes and regulations, the interest rate you get for your financing, and the specific fees required by the lender and the closing company (often a title company does the closing).

As a rough ballpark, closing costs will start in the neighborhood of a few thousand dollars, even for a $100,000 house. An appraisal by itself will often cost $500 or more. Your lender can provide their origination fee, closing costs, and your final prepaids based on the interest rate and date of your closing.

Grand Rounds by Dr. Tammy

Our jobs are stressful by nature. Having the home of your dreams can be the sanctuary you need at the end of the day, but don't overextend yourself so it adds to your stress. Budget for things like vacations, kids' educations, and even early retirement when you are deciding how much to spend on your new home. Burnout is real!

Chapter 2 Takeaways

 A mortgage is good debt because you are paying for an appreciating asset that can return more than you invested.

 You can still buy a house even if you have a big student loan debt balance. Understand your debt and what you need to do to pay it off and build that into your house-buying budget.

 Don't borrow the maximum the lender says you can. Decide for yourself what you are comfortable with and think about financial and life goals as part of your decision.

 Figure out the monthly house payment you are comfortable with and then work with a lender to determine how much house that can buy. Figure out your finances for yourself before you talk to a lender or a real estate agent or go looking at houses.

 Don't worry if you don't have enough cash for a down payment. With a physician loan, you don't need it. You will need cash for the closing costs, however.

 A big fancy house will not make you happy, but living paycheck-to-paycheck and working until you're 65 can make you very unhappy. Reward yourself with a nice house but balance that with other things in your life. Make getting your house paid off a goal before you reach 50 years old and look for a house that can help you do that. You'll be glad you did.

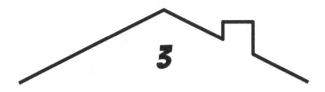

PHYSICIAN MORTGAGES—HOW THEY WORK AND WHY YOU SHOULD CONSIDER THEM

When you're ready to purchase a house, you have several options for obtaining financing, including all the loans available to people who are not physicians. These include conventional loans, government-backed loans such as VA (Veterans Administration) loans, FHA (Federal Housing Authority) loans, and USDA (United States Department of Agriculture) loans.

Plus, as a physician, you can take advantage of the special financing options some banks offer to you because of your profession—called a physician mortgage loan. With the exception of some physicians who are veterans, almost all others should seriously consider utilizing a physician mortgage loan.

All mortgages have the same basic components. However, there are a few distinct differences based on how mortgage loans are regulated, who guarantees ("backs") them, and who offers them. The basis for comparison is the *conventional loan*. A conventional loan is the most common mortgage option and it's available to everyone, regardless of profession.

Here's the basics of what you need for a conventional loan:

- A credit score of at least 620

- Proof of a stable income history

- A debt-to-income (DTI) ratio of 43% or less

- A down payment of at least 3-5% of the purchase price

- For less than 20% down, a conventional loan will charge private mortgage insurance (PMI)

- A requested loan amount of no more than $548,250 (this is the 2021 limit; this amount may be adjusted annually)

- For loan amounts above $548,250, new terms for what's called a *jumbo loan* will apply

Conventional loans are typically offered at very competitive interest rates, although these vary by lender. The rates offered for conventional loans should be your basis for comparing the interest rates of other types of loans, including physician loans.

For down payments of less than 20%, the PMI premium is added to the monthly payment. If you want to borrow more than $548,250, jumbo loans are typically offered at higher interest rates.

The terms for conventional loans are dictated by Fannie Mae (Federal National Mortgage Association, FNMA), the government-sponsored enterprise that guarantees conventional mortgage loans. Conventional loans are also called *secondary market loans* because they can be sold to multiple servicers and ultimately end up in mortgage-backed securities. It's common for lenders not to keep these loans, and lenders will sell them so they can remain liquid and continue to finance new loans (otherwise all their money would be tied up in existing loans).

Loan periods for any type of mortgage can vary from 10 to 30 years, with 30 years being a common one. The longer the loan period, the lower the combined principal and interest payment will be—and the more total interest you will pay over the life of the loan.

What Is a Physician Loan?

Lenders who offer physician mortgage loans treat you as a low-risk borrower and offer all the perks they would offer to someone who puts at least 20% down, without requiring that deposit. While conventional loans typically have the most competitive interest rates, physician mortgage loans can offer comparable rates without any money down and will still not charge you PMI. They may also loan you more than the conforming limit for conventional loans without additional fees. Lenders who specialize in physician loans treat physicians as valued and trusted customers.

Because physicians are highly paid, in demand, and typically want to borrow more money than the average homebuyer, it's lucrative for banks to offer these specialty loans. These lending institutions understand that physicians may not have money saved for a down payment due to the high cost of medical school, but they also know physicians are a good risk.

Physician loans are not guaranteed the same way conventional loans are because the issuing bank will hold the loan for its lifetime—they don't need Fannie Mae to guarantee them and they don't sell them. Because the bank will hold the loan in-house, physician loans are a type of *portfolio loan.*

Physician mortgage loans are customized, specialty loans and they don't have quite as many restrictions as conventional loans. The loan specifications are unique to the bank that issues them—so while what I'm describing is generally true for physician loans, make sure to verify their terms. Ask for each lender's *itemized fee sheet* so you clearly understand those terms. In addition, you want to know what other fees, such as an origination fee, they charge and the interest rate estimate they offer.

With that said, most physician loans generally offer the following terms and requirements to physicians:

- A good credit score (around 700)

- If you are a resident and have not yet started a new position, an offer letter will be accepted as proof of future income

- A down payment of 0% to 5%

- A debt-to-income ratio up to 45% (not including student loans, which are often ignored)

- Borrowing limits upward of $700,000

- They will offer 95% financing for loan amounts up to $1 million

- No PMI, regardless of the down payment amount

- They will allow you to close on a house before you start your first attending job, based on the offer letter

- If you are a resident, they evaluate income and credit score differently and give more leeway than conventional loans do

Physician loans are often offered at competitive interest rates, although every lender is different. You need to make a point of comparison shopping.

The three biggest reasons physician loans are a good idea are no PMI, no PMI, and no PMI—which means you can finance 100% of the loan amount. Outside of these loans, there are very limited options for 100% financing with other types of mortgages.

PHYSICIAN MORTGAGE LOAN = DOCTOR MORTGAGE LOAN

A physician mortgage loan and a doctor mortgage loan are the same thing and the terms are interchangeable. They may also be called physician home loans, physician loans, and doctor loans or possibly even professional's loan. They can also be offered to other healthcare professionals like dentists, pharmacists, attorneys, and optometrists.

Why Physicians Make Great Candidates for Mortgages

Why are physicians offered a product like a physician loan? As a resident, you don't have a big salary that would qualify you for a large mortgage. With the large amount of debt and possibly only a small amount of savings you may have, you may think there's no way you would qualify. So why the special treatment?

Lenders offer great benefits to physicians because medicine is a lucrative profession with strong demand. It's typically easy to find another job if you leave the one you're in. High salaries and steady employment represent low risk to lenders, so they are willing to offer you terms that benefit you but don't put them at too much risk.

But what about those student loans? Lenders know doctors have opportunities for loan forgiveness through various federal and state programs. Also, they can tell if you are responsible about paying your loans through your credit score. Physician loans generally require a credit score above 700, but this isn't usually a problem. You have likely been paying regularly on student loan debt for a while by the time you are ready to buy a house.

Doctors also statistically have lower default rates on loans than other types of borrowers. Some estimates state doctors have a 0.2% default rate, compared to the average consumer rate of more than 2%.

Ignoring your student loan debt and offering up to 100% financing with no PMI make it easier for physicians to get a mortgage loan. Let's take a closer look at the advantages and disadvantages of physician loans so you can make an educated decision about what's best for you.

Advantages and Disadvantages of Physician Mortgage Loans

One area where physician mortgage loans are no different from any other mortgage loan is this: you need to know what your own spending limits are. One of the biggest mistakes I see physicians make is buying such an expensive house that they find themselves living paycheck to paycheck. When they realize they want to make a change, they discover that the large debt is limiting their options in critical areas of their lives. Decide for yourself what's reasonable and don't buy a house that's twice as expensive as you originally were shopping for because you can get it for 0% down—or because the lender ignored your student. Use the benefits to put yourself in a better financial position, not a worse one.

Advantages

Most of these have already been mentioned, but here's more about why most physicians should seriously consider physician loans.

1. No or Low Down Payment

Buying a house with low or no money down is a tremendous benefit. Most mortgage products with 0% down come with big fees or specific requirements, and not many lenders offer this option at all. For many borrowers, coming up with a down payment is often the biggest hurdle to overcome and can take years.

And if you do have the cash for a down payment, instead of putting it toward the house, you can use it to pay your student loan debt, credit card debt, or increase your emergency fund. All of these alternative uses for your cash may be more beneficial to your finances than tying that money up in a house.

2. No PMI

Physician mortgages allow you to avoid PMI. Annual PMI costs are typically between 0.3% and 1.2% of the mortgage. With a conventional loan, you will pay this amount until you have paid off 20% of your mortgage. It can take years to reach this point.

Without PMI, your monthly payment will be smaller, allowing it to fit your budget better and leave more of your paycheck to go toward other expenses, rather than lining the pockets of a lender.

3. Strong Credit History Not Required

Don't worry about not having a long credit history, either. Most physicians don't, early in their careers. If you are not a first-time house buyer, the credit score requirements will be higher, likely 700 or above, which usually isn't a problem for most physicians.

4. Student Loans and Your Debt-to-Income (DTI) Ratio

While you've probably wished your student loans would disappear on their own, having them not factor into the financial equation could be the next best thing.

Many banks don't count your full standard payment on your student loans. They look only at what you are paying on your income-driven repayment. If you're in deferment or you're not paying on them yet, they don't count them in your debt.

Banks that look out for your best interests will count your loan payments when determining what you can borrow, but they may be more liberal with the debt ratio to make up for it. On a conventional loan, you qualify based on whether you got complete forbearance of your student loans. And if you are paying on them, you have to count a monthly 1% payment into what you qualify for.

Your debt-to-income ratio is extremely important because it's what lenders use to decide if an applicant is creditworthy. In most lending situations, lenders require you to have a DTI of 43% or less.

In a traditional lending situation, if you factored in the full payment on your student loans, you likely wouldn't qualify for a mortgage. With physician mortgage loans, the banks are aware that your loans could be well over six figures, but your future income outweighs the risk. Your other debts, however—credit cards, lines of credit, vehicle loans, etc.—will all count toward your DTI.

5. Exempt From Caps on Loans

Most borrowers have limits on how much money they can borrow. There are also additional fees if they go above the limit and have to get a jumbo loan. Jumbo loans are loans for more than the "conforming limit" of $548,250 (in 2021) for a conventional mortgage. While jumbo loans are not guaranteed by Fannie Mae, they may still be called a conventional loan. They will likely have more stringent credit score requirements and may also require a higher interest rate.

For physician loans, some banks do change their rates and possibly their down payment requirements, depending on the size of the loan. But for others, you can put 0% down on any size loan and the interest rate may not change. Shop around with different lenders and ask questions.

Disadvantages

The downside of any loan is that lenders will often offer to lend you significantly more money than you need. It can be enticing to see that letter qualifying you for *X* dollars when you are shopping for something in *Y* range. You need to do what's right for you. Figure out your budget and stick with it.

Before you agree to take on a physician loan, carefully consider all the pros and cons for these types of mortgages.

1. Most Physician Mortgages Have Variable Interest Rates

Many lenders for physician loans will quote you a variable interest rate instead of a fixed interest rate. Ask potential lenders what they offer when you interview them. Whether a variable-rate loan is a good choice for you largely depends on two things: whether you will be staying in the house long term and how the initial period rate on the variable loan compares to current fixed rates. You'll find more on fixed- and variable-rate loans in the next chapter.

2. Physician Mortgages May Have Higher Interest Rates

Lenders who provide physician home loans often extend the same interest rates as they would to a jumbo loan, which typically require a higher interest rate than a conventional loan. But with some lenders, the interest rates are no higher than conventional rates. So the real caveat here is to find the right lender.

Lenders don't charge PMI on physician loans, and some lenders will make up for that lost income from PMI by charging higher interest rates. The difference might be around 0.25%.

Each bank has its own set of rules and regulations, and also its own interest rates. One bank may charge as much as a full percentage point difference for a physician loan versus a conventional loan. These interest rate differences add up significantly over time.

For instance, if you buy a $250,000 home with 0% down, a 3.75% interest rate, and a 30-year term, you'll pay $179,673 total in interest. Compare that to a 3.5% interest rate over 30 years, where the total interest is $154,140. That's $25,000 in additional interest you'll pay—essentially 10% of what you borrowed initially. There are two caveats: the difference will be less if you don't stay in that house for 30 years or if you pay off the loan in less than 30 years.

Another option, if you need the benefits of a physician mortgage loan but are unable to find one with a competitive interest rate, is you can always re-finance a physician mortgage loan into a conventional mortgage once you've built up 20% equity or more. Refinancing is not free (there are several fees involved) but can be a viable option later on, if interest rates drop.

A few other factors also affect your interest rate. Some of them you can use to your benefit, and others are out of your control.

Your credit score has quite a bit to do with the rate you'll be quoted. The better your credit score, the better your rates. So if you are not yet ready to buy a house, in the meantime the best thing you can do to save yourself money when you are ready is pay your bills on time and pay down your debt.

Shopping multiple lenders may be the most important thing you can do to help your rates. Amazingly, even for a big purchase like a home, most people never shop around for a lender. Even if you're pressed for time, get comparison quotes. You could save yourself thousands in interest just by talking to more than one lender.

The economy and the actions of the Federal Reserve Bank are also big fac-tors in where interest rates are—and those end up being part of "the market" and are out of your control. If you are researching your options ahead of time, you can watch to see if rates are increasing or decreasing.

3. Limitations with Condos and Primary Residence Requirements

If you are thinking about purchasing a condo, make sure your lender will allow you to use a physician mortgage loan for this purpose.

Most lenders for doctor loans will not finance a condo, including non-warrantable condos, due to the higher risk they pose for the lender.

Furthermore, physician mortgages can only be used for your primary residence. You typically can't use these loans to purchase vacation or rental properties.

4. Higher Fees

Physician loans may also have higher fees than conventional loans in terms of closing costs. As I keep saying, fees and many other aspects of the loan vary with different lenders. Always ask your lender for a breakdown of fees, which they will put in an itemized fee sheet. You can also ask for a comparison of fees, interest rates, and qualification amounts for a physician loan versus a conventional loan to see which is better for you.

5. It Takes Longer to Build Up Equity

Zero down payment is certainly an attractive offer. The downside is it will take you a few years to build equity in your house. The housing market crash of 2008 and the related Great Recession are still fresh in many people's minds, and those with little equity in their houses at the time suffered serious consequences, especially if they also lost their income.

It is harder to sell a home when you haven't built up equity. If you need as much money as possible from the sale, it may be more difficult to put money into renovations, staging, or real estate agent fees.

The biggest financial risk to having no equity in your house comes if you need to sell quickly. Often quick equates to a lower price. This happens for many reasons: job changes, divorce, or even a move to a better school district.

What Else?

Understand all of your options before committing to a physician mortgage. Make sure the physician mortgage loan is your best option.

If you can afford a 20% down payment on the loan amount you want, you may get a better deal on a conventional loan. You will still avoid PMI and if you have that kind of cash handy to put down, you likely have a credit score good enough to qualify for the best interest rates.

If you qualify for a VA loan (more on that in the next chapter), that will likely have better terms than either the conventional or the physician loan. So keep this in mind if you are a veteran.

HIPPOCRATIC HOUSE CHECKLIST

Documents You Will Need for a Physician Loan Application

If you are a wage earner and not a business owner, you'll need these things:

- ☐ Two years' worth of W2s
- ☐ Two recent pay stubs
- ☐ Two years' worth of tax returns
- ☐ Two months' worth of bank statements
- ☐ Most recent retirement account statement
- ☐ Copy of your medical license

If you are self-employed, you will need to provide information on two years' worth of income to show your income is steady and preferably increasing.

If you are not a U.S. citizen, ask your lender what documentation they need. They may require a green card or possibly a J-1 visa.

HIPPOCRATIC HOUSE CHECKLIST

Is a Physician Mortgage Right for You?

Here are some circumstances that can make a physician mortgage a great choice for financing your first home purchase:

- ☐ You don't have a lot of cash for a down payment—less than 3% of the purchase price.
- ☐ Including your student loan payments and your new mortgage, your debt-to-income ratio will be below 45%.
- ☐ Your credit score is at least 700 if you are an attending.
- ☐ You want to borrow more than the conforming limit for conventional loans—which is $548,250 in 2021.

If you have enough cash for 20% down plus your closing costs, and it's important to you to have equity in your house from the beginning *and* you are planning to borrow less than the conforming limit, you may get a lower interest rate on a conventional loan than you would on a physician loan—but that depends on the lender you choose.

If you have enough cash for 20% down, you should definitely get an itemized fee sheet for a conventional loan as well as a physician loan from at least two lenders, so you can be sure you get the best deal.

Grand Rounds by Dr. Tammy

It doesn't feel like we get many perks anymore for being physicians, but a physician loan can be one of the best. Banks want our business because we pay our debts. Docs can get a new home with no money down at several banks. If you've saved 20% down for your home, that's wonderful, but you can also apply that money toward loans with higher interest rates, keep it in an emergency fund, or invest it if you find something with a better rate of return than your home will cost you. As a doc, you have options most people don't have.

Chapter 3 Takeaways

 Physician mortgage loans are customized products created by the banks that offer them, and the terms can vary. Be sure to ask for a fee sheet so you understand the terms.

 The main advantages physician loans offer over conventional financing are these:

- Financing up to 100% of the purchase price
- No PMI, even with 0% down payment
- The option of borrowing more than the conventional financing conforming limit at competitive interest rates and with no PMI
- Loan approval based on future income for residents in the form of an offer letter, even before you start the job (you can't do this with any other kind of financing)

 Because physician loans give you the option of financing 100% of the home you want to buy, you can use your savings in other ways that benefit your financial bottom line:

- Paying off high-interest consumer debt
- Paying off student loans
- Building your emergency fund
- Investments

 A real physician mortgage loan will not charge PMI. If you are quoted PMI, keep looking to see if you can find a better option.

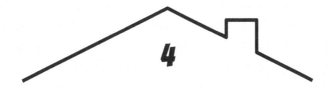

MORTGAGE BASICS AND OTHER MORTGAGE OPTIONS

A mortgage is a loan specifically for buying a house, and the house itself acts as the collateral for the loan. As long as you make timely mortgage payments, you own the house. If at some point you can't make the payments, the bank takes your house and sells it to cover the debt (this process is called foreclosure). Lenders don't want to go into foreclosure; they want you to make the payments.

Lenders evaluate each borrower in terms of their ability to reliably pay back the debt as agreed. The greater the perceived risk, the more expensive the lending terms will be, in terms of interest rate charged and possibly private mortgage insurance (PMI), which the borrower must pay for the benefit of the lender.

You'll get better terms for conventional loans if you can put at least 20% of the purchase price down. This is the basis for how conventional mortgage loans are set up. The best financing terms are available to those with good credit scores who can put 20% or more down—those borrowers will pay less interest and won't have to pay for PMI.

Many people don't realize how much of the mortgage loan procurement process is negotiable. They also don't realize how much lenders' fees and rates can vary.

> Shopping for a mortgage lender is as important as shopping for the house itself.

Physicians are considered by lenders to be a much lower lending risk than other individuals. Physicians also typically want a larger house and a larger loan than the average borrower, making specialized loans that target physicians a lucrative strategy for lenders.

While a physician mortgage is a great option for almost all physicians, other types of loans might offer better terms if you qualify for them. Make sure you investigate other options and compare.

Conventional Mortgage Loans: The Baseline

Conventional mortgage requirements were mentioned in the previous chapter for comparison purposes because conventional financing is the most common type of mortgage.

A conventional mortgage has these basic requirements, based on Fannie Mae guidelines:

1. Require payment of PMI if you put down less than 20%
2. A loan limit of $548,250 (in 2021) or increased interest rates for a jumbo loan above that amount
3. Require recent pay stubs as proof of employment and income
4. Require a debt-to-income (DTI) ratio of 43% or less

It's possible to obtain a conventional mortgage with as little as 3-5% down, however they will always charge PMI.

Private Mortgage Insurance (PMI) in More Detail

PMI is an insurance policy that benefits the lender and protects them against the risk that you will default on your home loan. You (the buyer, the borrower) have to pay for PMI if it is required, but it benefits only the lender. PMI is offered by third-party insurance companies that are willing to share the risk with the lender.

Conventional loans require that you pay for PMI until you reach 20% equity, however long that takes.

Terminology: Equity, Down Payments, and Loan-to-Value Ratio

A 20% down payment is a magic number for conventional financing; if you can put down 20% or more, the loan terms will be better and the cost of borrowing will be less—and you won't have to pay for PMI. You will then be borrowing 80% of the house purchase price.

Lenders use the term "loan-to-value" (LTV) ratio or percentage to express how much is being borrowed in a different way—if you make a 20% down payment on a house, the loan-to-value ratio is 80%. If you put 0% down, the loan to value is 100%. The lower the LTV, the less risk a lender places on that loan, and the better terms you will get.

If you put down 20% on a house purchase, you have 20% equity in that house immediately after the closing, when they hand you the keys.

Jumbo Loans

Jumbo loans are conventional mortgage loans for amounts above the limits set by Fannie Mae. Designed to finance luxury properties and homes in highly competitive local real estate markets, jumbo mortgages come with unique underwriting requirements and tax implications.

In comparison to a conventional loan, a jumbo loan requires a higher income, higher credit scores, and enough assets to cover 6-12 months' worth of mortgage payments. A lower credit score can potentially be offset with a lower debt-to-income ratio. Down payment requirements are typically 10-20%.

A lender offering physician mortgages will usually not change the interest rate or other terms for loan amounts above the conventional limit, and this is one of the advantages of a physician mortgage over a conventional mortgage. However, you should always ask the question about higher loan amounts because every lender has their own terms for physician mortgages.

What's in a Mortgage Payment?

Mortgage payments have two basic components: principal and interest (P&I). The *principal* is the actual amount of money that you borrow and have to pay back. Think of *interest* as the fee you pay to the lender in exchange for their lending you the principal needed to purchase the house.

Each monthly principal payment reduces the balance on the loan while the interest payment is paying the cost of the loan. The first few years of mortgage payments contribute little toward the principal and more toward the interest—the combined total will remain constant over the life of a loan for a fixed interest loan, but the initial ratio puts more toward interest and this shifts to contributing more toward the principal as the years go by.

Your mortgage payment will also usually include taxes and insurance.

Anatomy of a Mortgage Payment

1. Principal: The amount that goes toward paying down your loan balance.
2. Interest: The fee you pay to the lender for borrowing money.
3. Property taxes: Your annual property taxes will be estimated, and 1/12th of that amount will be added to your monthly payment and held in escrow until payment is due.
4. Homeowners insurance: Your lender will require you to carry homeowners insurance. Like property taxes, 1/12th of the annual insurance premium will be added to your monthly payment and held in escrow until payment is due.

In some areas and housing developments, the homeowners association (HOA) dues may be treated like taxes and insurance and added to your mortgage payment, if those fees are significant. This is more common in high cost of living areas and condominium or patio home developments where maintenance is high.

What Is Escrow?

An escrow account is an account set up by a third party to hold funds for future payments or for a transaction. An escrow account is used to hold the earnest money a buyer puts up as part of their offer on a piece of real estate.

A slightly different type of escrow account is set up by the loan processing company to hold the portion of the funds from your monthly mortgage payments that will go toward paying taxes and homeowners insurance. Some of the "prepaids" portion of your cash required at closing will go toward the initial funding of that escrow account, as required by the mortgage company.

Most people who have mortgages have an escrow account with the loan servicing company for taxes and insurance. So, whenever you set up an escrow account, the bank wants to have a reserve so that next year when your bill comes due, they have enough money to pay your taxes and insurance, plus a cushion of a couple of months' worth of payments. The amount required for taxes and insurance is reevaluated every year and your payment adjusted to accommodate that change. It can be an increase or a decrease.

Mortgage Interest Rates

Lenders can adjust interest rates they offer based on their policies and their evaluation of you as a borrower. The interest rate you must pay on your loan significantly affects how much house you can afford. Do a simple comparison between 3%, 4%, and 5% interest rates using a mortgage calculator to see what happens to the total principal and interest. Interest rates in the U.S. have been hovering in the range of 3-4% for most of the late 2010s and into the 2020s, but markets change constantly. It's worth shopping for the most competitive rate you can find in the current market.

Interest rates in the U.S. are affected by government policies. For fixed-rate mortgages, interest rates follow the 10-year bond market. Fannie Mae sets the size limit for conventional mortgages and evaluates those values each year to adjust for market changes. In 2019, the conventional loan limit was $484,350 for most areas of the country, except for high-cost areas like Hawaii and Alaska, where it was set at $726,525. In 2020, the conventional loan limit was increased to $510,400 and to $765,600 for high-cost areas. In 2021, the limit was $548,250 and up to $822,375 in high-cost areas.

Your lender can keep you updated on current interest rates and advise you on the best loan type for your circumstances. When you are shopping for lenders, ask each one you talk to for an itemized fee sheet showing their standard fees and current interest rate for the kind of mortgage you are considering.

Mortgages are offered for different borrowing periods and as either fixed interest rate or variable interest rate loans that adjust with the market rates. Which one works best for you depends on your circumstances and what's happening with the interest rate market and economy at the time you secure the loan.

Fixed-Rate Loans

A fixed interest rate loan will have the same interest rate throughout the life of the loan. It will not be subject to market fluctuations or any other outside factors. A fixed-rate loan is a great way to lock into a low rate and is easy to budget for.

Fixed-rate loans are available for periods of time between 10 and 30 years. The shorter the period of time, the lower the interest rate will be. The most common time periods are 15 and 30 years.

A great way for a physician to get started in homeownership would be to finance a house they can afford with a 15-year loan so they can look forward to being debt-free by the time they are 45 or so. While the monthly payment will be higher for a 15-year loan than a 30-year loan, you'll save thousands in reduced interest.

Interest Rate Comparisons on 15- and 30-Year Fixed-Rate Mortgages

The following chart shows the comparison of P&I payments for 15- and 30-year fixed-rate mortgages at $500,000.

	Monthly P&I Payment	
Interest Rate	15 Years	30 Years
3%	$3,453	$2,108
4%	$3,698	$2,387
5%	$3,954	$2,684

Effect of loan term on principal and interest payments for fixed interest rates on a $500,000 mortgage loan.

A fixed-rate loan is great if you plan to stay in your house as long as possible. You'll lock in your rate and won't have to worry about the payment changing from one year to the next.

If interest rates go below the rate you are paying after you purchase your house, you could consider refinancing your remaining loan balance. For a refinance to make sense (give you a return on the closing costs you will have to pay in a reasonable amount of time), interest rates need to be significantly lower than you are current paying—say at least 0.5%—and you should do the same cost-benefit calculation as described below for buying points to lower your interest rate. This is done by dividing the monthly savings into the total closing costs to find your break-even point in months.

My standard rule is if you don't break even on the cost of the refinance in three and a half years or less, it's not worth doing—too expensive for what you get.

Adjustable-Rate Loans

The main alternative to the fixed-rate mortgage is a type of variable-rate loan called the adjustable-rate mortgage (ARM). With this loan, the interest rate will change after a fixed initial period. This is a common option for physician mortgage loans. Some lenders only offer adjustable-rate physician loans.

An ARM is a combination of a fixed-rate and an adjustable-rate loan. For instance, a 5/1 30-year ARM offers a fixed interest rate for the first five years of the loan, and then the rate will adjust once a year for the remaining 25 years. If interest rates are going up, your payment could continue to increase over the years—or it could go down if rates go down. Most ARMs include a limit on how much the interest rate can increase each year (called a cap), such as no more than a 2% increase, for example.

The most common adjustable-rate option is the 5/1 loan, but you can also find mortgages with 3/1, 7/1, and 10/1 ARM options.

ARMs can be a good option especially for residents, if they want to buy a house for their residency and sell it when their residency is over. ARMs typically have a lower interest rate during the initial period than a fixed-rate loan will, especially if interest rates are trending upward.

Because the interest rate and therefore your monthly payment can change every year after the fixed rate period, ARMs can be difficult to budget for. The change in payment could be minimal or it could be significant, depending on the market.

The 10/1 loan is one of the best ARMs to consider because many people don't stay in a house longer than 10 years anyway—even if they bought it thinking it was their forever home. Another option is to pay the house off early, within that time.

However, always compare interest rates on an ARM to the current fixed rates to make sure you get the best deal. The 10/1 and even 15/1 ARMs may not offer a lower interest rate for the fixed initial period than a simple fixed-rate loan. It depends on what the market is doing. To be worth the risk of that adjustable rate, you should expect to save at least 0.5% on the initial interest rate to take on an ARM rather than a fixed-rate loan. You may be better off to simply get a 15-year or 30-year fixed-rate loan and pay it off ahead of time.

When Are ARMS a Good Deal?

To evaluate an ARM in comparison to a fixed-rate option, first compare the interest rate of fixed-rate mortgages to the initial fixed period of the ARM rate you are offered.

If rates are trending upward, ARMs may offer lower initial rates than the fixed-rate products. Rates change all the time, so when you are shopping, monitor mortgage interest rates so you know if they are trending up or down.

Your lender can also advise you what is your best move in the current market conditions. ARMs can be a good option, especially if you think you will either want to move and sell the house before the fixed rate period expires or refinance the loan to a fixed rate.

In the early 2000s, you could get ARMs with an initial rate of 2.5% when the fixed rate was 5%. Always look closely at the terms on ARMs (the caps) so you know what the worst case might be, if interest rates start to increase.

Purchasing Points to Lower the Interest Rate

You may have heard of people buying "points" when they finance or refinance a house. A point is 1% of the loan amount and is used as a fee to "buy" a lower interest rate for the life of the loan. They may also be used for other fees. So if you are borrowing $500,000 and are charged a point for the loan, that point costs $5,000. Typically one point will reduce the interest rate by one-quarter percent (0.25%). Points are paid as part of the closing costs, in cash.

Most lenders offer discount points to reduce the interest rate, however in many cases this is not money well spent. For example, if the rate is 3.5% for a loan amount of $500,000, typically paying a point would reduce the rate 0.25% to 3.25% on a 30-year fixed rate. And most lenders, if they do offer points, would cap the number of points you can buy at two—so the most you could lower your rate would be 0.5%, in this example. If you buy one point, your cost benefit would be $50 a month at a cost of $5,000. You wouldn't break even on that expense (saving $50 per month) until after your 100th payment—eight and one-third years. This is too long, in my opinion. This wouldn't be worth doing unless you were certain you will stay in the house for a long time, so you can reap some benefit from that reduced rate.

Take a close look at the cost and benefit of buying points before you decide to do it. While shopping different lenders for the lowest interest rate you can find is worth the effort, paying additional money to lower your interest rate by a small amount may not be a money-saving move.

Calculate the Time to Break Even

To calculate how many payments and how much time will pass before you break even on the expense of buying points, take your monthly savings and divide that number into the cost of the point(s). That's the number of payments you will have to make before you begin to save any money. For the above example, with 100 payments—which is over eight years—you might be better off putting that $5,000 into your emergency fund or investing it.

> **Buying points to lower your interest rate is usually not a good investment.**

Points often don't work out to be a good investment because if you decide to sell the house or refinance before you reach the break-even point, you don't save anything and you're out $5,000. You don't know what will happen within eight years. My personal rule is this: it's not worth investing money on points if you won't get your money back in 42 months—three and a half years. Any longer than that and it's not worth the gamble.

This is the same thought process you should use to decide if it's worth it to refinance. If it costs $4,000 to refinance, then it better save at least $100 a month. If you won't break even on the cost versus the benefit in 42 months, I advise you not to do it. Many lenders won't ask those questions or help you with the risk versus benefit calculation.

Interest Rates on Fixed-Rate Mortgage Loans

When you request a loan from your lender, that lender is borrowing money based on current market rates—for whatever the loan period is, up to 30 years. When they offer a fixed rate for the length of the loan, they are effectively locking an interest rate. The longer the loan period, the more expensive it is to borrow money—and the higher the interest rate will be. That's why the interest rate is higher for a 30-year fixed rate than a 15-year fixed rate, no matter what the market is doing.

Locking Rates Before Closing

When you go through the preapproval process, you will be quoted a current interest rate for the type of loan you are considering, but that is not a guaranteed rate. Most lenders require that you have a property "under contract"—that is, you've made an offer on a house and the seller has accepted it, and you have negotiated the price and other contingency details and both have signed—before you can request a lock. The rate goes with the property.

Once you have a house under contract, a series of required steps are set in motion that culminate with the closing date that officially makes you the owner of the house. One of those steps is locking your interest rate. You don't have to lock a rate until you are within the last 10 days or so before closing. You can't wait until the last day to lock the rate because it takes time to finalize the loan.

The most common interest rate lock period is 30 days. It's typical for this lock to expire in 30 days, unless you ask for a longer period of time. The rate lock commitment fee will cost more for longer lock periods (if your closing won't be for 45 or 90 days, for example), or else you will pay a higher interest rate. The lock fee may be an up-front fee or added to your closing costs.

Many borrowers assume the interest rate they will pay is either what it was the day they applied for the loan or the day they close. But it's neither. It's locked whenever you request the rate lock, and you should then get a *loan estimate* or a *rate lock commitment* notice showing that your rate is locked. Don't assume your rate is locked at the time you apply for a loan. We've included a blank example loan estimate form (multiple pages) that you can access at DougCrouse.com.

Other Loan Options: FHA, USDA, and VA Loans

FHA, USDA, and VA loans are government-backed loans with specific qualification requirements. With the exception of VA loans, if you qualify for a conventional or a physician mortgage, these will be better options for you than FHA or USDA loans. While some of the terms for these loans look attractive, they come with added fees and limitations that may make them unattractive for many physicians. These three loan types are insured by the U.S. government.

FHA loans are a good option for people with low credit scores, but otherwise a conventional loan or a physician loan will generally offer better terms. FHA loans also have a lower conforming limit for the loan amount than conventional loans. USDA loans have income restrictions for eligibility and also regional restrictions—housing must be in designated rural areas.

FHA Loans

FHA loan interest rates are negotiable and are based on the current market, so they tend to be at lower interest rates than conventional financing. This sounds good, but it comes at a cost because FHA loans require mortgage insurance (through the U.S. government) *for the life of the loan,* not just until the buyer has 20% equity. And that PMI will normally cost twice as much as PMI for a conventional loan. There is also an additional PMI charge of 1.75% that must be paid up front with the closing costs. So FHA loan terms are not as good as the lower interest rate might lead you to believe.

Typically, conventional loans are available for people with a score of 620 or higher, but FHA loans require only a 580 credit score. FHA loans will allow you to have a debt ratio of 55% of your gross income, much higher than a physician loan will allow.

An FHA loan requires 3.5% down instead of the 20% for a conventional loan, and that 3.5% could be a gift from family. The credit score requirement drops even lower (to 500) if you make at least a 10% down payment. With these requirements, many people assume the FHA loan is only for first-time borrowers, but you can qualify for an FHA loan at any time, even if you have previously owned a home.

FHA loans have limits on the size of the loan based on the geographical area (called the market service area or MSA). Typically they are 70% of the conventional loan limit. For instance, in Kansas City, the FHA loan limit in 2021 was $356,362. That would buy a nice house in Kansas City at that time, but it may not be what a physician is looking for. In California, the financing limit might be over $800,000 based on what they consider "affordable."

The biggest drawback to the FHA loan is the upfront PMI charge of 1.75%, in addition to the monthly PMI. They are considered riskier loans, and in some markets may be quite expensive to get.

FHA loans are not a better option than either conventional loans or physician loans unless you don't meet the credit requirements for a physician loan or a conventional loan.

USDA Loans

USDA loans are offered in specifically designated rural and suburban areas only, to lower- and middle-income borrowers. Interest rates tend to be very competitive and PMI charges are much less than for FHA loans. They also offer 100% financing options. They are available to first-time homebuyers but are not limited to that group. Residents may qualify for the income requirements, but the typical physician salary will disqualify you from eligibility for USDA loans. Borrowing limits range from $300,000 to $400,000, depending on income. Visit the Resources page for a link to more information about USDA loans.

VA Loans

VA (Veterans Administration) loans are offered to military veterans, and the terms for these are often better than you can obtain any other way, especially if you have a qualifying disability. So if you qualify, get quotes on a VA loan for comparison with other options you want to explore.

Veterans Administration loans were designed for members of the military and their spouses. Although the government is not the lender for a VA loan, a certain percentage of the loan is backed by the government. This makes it an attractive product for both the borrower and the lender.

Hands down, the best mortgage option—whether you're a physician or not—is the VA loan. Similar to the physician mortgage loan, the VA loan does not require a down payment and you will not be charged for PMI either. The interest rates on VA loans are very competitive and similar to conventional loans. However, only veterans of the U.S. military or their spouses qualify.

These are the general qualifying criteria:

- Active-duty service in any branch of the armed forces for a minimum of 90 consecutive days during wartime, or

- Active-duty service in any branch of the armed forces for a minimum of 181 days of active duty during peacetime, or

- Service in any branch of the armed forces for more than six years in the National Guard or reserves, or

- You are the spouse of a military member who died while on active duty or as the result of a service-connected disability, and who has not remarried.

You do not need to have the eligibility certificate in hand to reach out to a lender or to prequalify. Check the Resources section in this book for a link to the VA eligibility requirements.

Benefits of a VA Loan

Here is a summary of the benefits of VA mortgage loans:

- **No or low down payment:** You can finance for up to 100% of the purchase price.

- **No PMI:** VA loans do not require borrowers to carry PMI.

- **Flexibility:** Once you have built up some equity, you have access to use that equity toward future lines of credit to finance renovations or purchase another house, if you wish. This is a unique benefit of VA loans.

- **No income requirement to qualify:** There is no minimum income requirement to qualify for the VA loan, however you will obviously be expected to have enough income to cover your mortgage payment and other monthly expenses. The bank will calculate this when you submit your application. This is especially helpful if you are a resident and don't have a high salary yet.

You can use any lender you wish to provide a loan as long as they are a VA-approved lender. You do not need to find a lender that only works with the military.

The main difference between physician loans and VA loans is the VA loans are a formalized product requiring documentation of military status or association, whereas physician loans simply require a letter of employment verification, just as any conventional loan would.

Can I Qualify for Both a Physician Loan and a VA Loan?

Perhaps you are a veteran and a physician at the same time. VA loan interest rates typically run 0.25-0.5% lower than a physician loan, but VA loans have an additional funding fee of 2.15-3.3% up front, so they are fairly equal in cost to a physician loan.

If you have the choice between a VA loan and a physician mortgage, a VA loan will almost always be the better choice, especially if you have a VA-related disability. If you have 10% disability (or more), you're exempt from the VA funding fee, which is essentially the equivalent of a one-time PMI payment. VA loans use the same conforming limits as conventional loans ($548,250 for most regions in 2021), however you should ask about this, as the rules can change based on legislation. Also, these numbers tend to go up because as housing costs go up, so do lending limits.

How to Choose a Loan

For most physicians, a physician loan provides the most benefits with competitive terms. Before you start the preapproval process, discuss your loan options with your lender and use the following guidelines as a starting point for your decision. You must choose a specific loan type to go forward with the preapproval process.

1. **Choose the Loan Type**

   a. If your credit score is good and you have a 20% down payment, compare conventional loans against physician loans. The conventional loan may offer the best interest rate and you won't have to pay PMI.

b. If you qualify for a VA loan, definitely look into these as they may give you the best terms of all.

c. If your credit score is too low for physician loans and conventional loans and you don't qualify for a VA loan, look at FHA and USDA loans.

2. **Determine Length of the Loan**

a. Plug numbers into a mortgage calculator to compare fixed-rate loans at 15 and 30 years to determine if you can handle the higher monthly payments of a 15-year mortgage. Use these numbers as a baseline estimate of your monthly payments.

b. Consider buying a little less house so you can go with a 15-year mortgage—the personal and financial benefits to having your home paid off before you reach the age of 50 cannot be underestimated.

c. A 30-year mortgage is also a good option, especially if you set up your budget to make extra payments so you can pay it off early.

3. **Compare Fixed-Rate to Adjustable-Rate Loans**

a. Compare interest rates on fixed rate and 5/1, 7/1, or 10/1 ARMs to see if the initial rate on the ARMs is lower.

b. When rates are trending upward, ARMs become worth the risk if the initial rate period for the ARM is significantly below the fixed-rate loan.

4. **Verify No Prepayment Penalty**

a. Always ask if there is a prepayment penalty with any mortgage. If there is one, find out the details and consider carefully if the loan has benefits to offset this disadvantage. You should be able to find a lender who does not include a prepayment penalty in their terms.

Never Forget That a Mortgage Is Debt

While a home mortgage is considered "good" debt and necessary debt, it is still debt and a liability. A mortgage is not something you should always have, contrary to popular belief. You can pay it off ahead of schedule if you plan for it.

More on Fixed- Versus Adjustable-Rate Loans

For someone who stays in a house long term, the adjustable (or variable) rate might be stressful. But if you will only be in the home for five to seven years, an ARM can be a great option if the initial interest rate period of the ARM is lower than a fixed-rate loan.

Residents will almost always be better off taking an adjustable-rate mortgage with a lower rate than the fixed, knowing they will sell that house in five years.

How fixed- and adjustable-rate mortgages compare changes with the market. Interest rates on ARMs are not always lower than fixed-rate loans.

Example: If you could get a 30-year fixed at 3.5% or you could get a 5/1 ARM at 3%, and you know you will be selling that house within five years, you're leaving money on the table by not taking the ARM. Take the lower interest rate because you know you'll sell it at the end of four years anyway. Then you'll save 0.5% times four years. As a rough estimate for an interest rate of 2%, if you bought a $200,000 house, you just saved $4-5,000.

HIPPOCRATIC HOUSE CHECKLIST

Know Your Numbers

Make sure you know your numbers so you can choose the right loan product for you:

- ❑ Competitive interest rates for the current market (conventional mortgage rates are a good place to start).

- ❑ Your credit score: A score of 700 (with some wiggle room between 680 and 750) is generally okay. Don't let a lower score stop you from reaching out to discuss your situation with a lender. You can likely still qualify for a loan at a similar or only slightly more expensive rate.

- ❑ The maximum mortgage payment you are willing to commit to monthly.

- ❑ The maximum house price you are willing to pay (get guidance from your lender on this).

- ❑ Closing costs for a physician loan (ask your lender for a quote).

- ❑ Closing costs for a comparable conventional loan (ask for a quote).

- ❑ Debt-to-income ratio (DTI): Most lenders look for a DTI of 45% or less, not including your student loans. It's always a good idea to keep debt low, but that ratio specifically means you should not be using more than 45% of your available credit.

HIPPOCRATIC HOUSE CHECKLIST

Which Loan Is Best?

You need to choose a loan type and length as well as a fixed or adjustable interest rate as part of your preapproval process. That information will be in your offer contract as a finance contingency, along with a maximum interest rate you will finance for—so if the market jumps and you can't get the interest rate you wanted and the loan becomes unaffordable, you have an out.

The best loan product is the one that works for your circumstances. The major differentiators for which type will work best for you are these:

1. **Your credit score:**

   ❑ Above 700 and any loan type is available to you, at the best rates.

   ❑ 620-700+ will qualify you for conventional loans.

   ❑ Below 620 will require you to look at VA loans if you are a veteran or FHA or USDA loans if you are not a veteran.

2. **Your veteran status and disability status:**

   ❑ You must be a veteran of the U.S. military to qualify for a VA loan.

   ❑ An unbeatable combination is veteran status with a veteran-related 10% or more disability to qualify you for a VA loan and waive the funding fee.

3. **Your cash reserves:**

   ❑ If you have 20% down and are not a veteran, a physician loan or a conventional loan are both great options.

   ❑ If you don't have a down payment or want to use your money for other purposes, a VA loan or a physician loan will likely offer the best terms.

4. **Your monthly budget:**

   ❑ If you have the monthly cash flow, consider a 15-year mort-gage. You will save a significant amount in interest over the life of that shorter loan. Owning your house outright in 15 years frees you to consider many alternatives to working full time until you're 65.

5. **Your life plans:**

   ❑ If you know you will likely be moving in five to seven years, consider an ARM if the initial period interest rate is lower than fixed-rate mortgages.

The typical reason a physician might not qualify for a physician mortgage is bad credit, which then pushes them toward the conventional or FHA, VA, and USDA loans, which are more forgiving on credit.

Grand Rounds by Dr. Tammy

Doug and I have purchased three homes since we've been together. We used a conventional loan for a home when I was still in med school, a portfolio loan at a small local bank for a unique home on acreage, and a physician loan for our current house. We plan to have the house paid off in less than five years, so we chose an ARM to get the very best interest rate.

There are so many options. You need a mortgage banker who is familiar with all the options, someone who is honest and will tell you if their product is not the right one for you. Bonus points for the lender who will refer you to the right person or bank for your needs! It's also helpful to have a lender who will be available when you need them in the evenings and on weekends, not just Monday through Friday from 8 to 5.

Chapter 4 Takeaways

 Conventional mortgage financing is a good comparison benchmark for other types of loans and is the most common type of financing offered in the U.S. They usually offer competitive interest rates and the best terms for borrowers who can pay a 20% down payment.

 For any mortgage loan, the longer the loan period, the lower the monthly principal and interest payment will be—and the more total interest you will pay over the life of the loan.

 If your credit score is 700 or better, for most physicians, the only reason you would want to consider anything other than a physician mortgage (if you don't have 20% down) is if you qualify for a VA loan.

 If you have the 20% down payment, you'll want to compare conventional or jumbo conventional loans with the physician loan terms to make sure you're getting the best deal.

 A conventional loan will have only very limited options for 100% financing and they will come with higher expenses. USDA loans allow it and VA loans allow it, and some other down payment assistance programs may allow it. This is a huge benefit with physician loans.

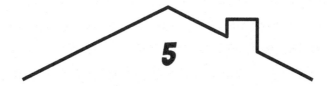

CHOOSING A LENDER AND GETTING PREAPPROVED

How to Find a Lender

Seek out at least two to four potential lenders who work solely with physicians or who focus on physicians. These will most likely be mortgage bankers. Personal recommendations from colleagues and friends are a great place to start.

The best physician mortgage loans are geared generally toward doctors who have completed their residency, and not as much toward residents, fellows, or medical students. That is tied to the fact that qualifying for a mortgage loan typically requires a steady income.

However, even as a resident, you can find physician loans that work for your situation. Once you determine that you are ready to buy a house, reach out to some lenders. Consultations will cost you about an hour of your time.

Look at More Than Interest Rates

Getting a good interest rate is important, but there are several questions you'll want to ask when you speak with a potential lender. Use the method described in chapter 2 to know what you can afford in terms of a monthly house payment before you start talking with lenders. The calculations they use to determine what they will lend to you are a maximum based on the risk that you will default—which has nothing to do with your comfort level or other financial goals.

Lender Interview: Questions to Ask

No matter what kind of loan you are considering, ask these questions to clarify what is being offered. Because physician loans are customized products offered by individual banks, you need to make sure you understand what the terms and fees will be.

1. Do you do business in my geographic region?

    Many lenders you work with will not be local to you. Bank regulations vary by state and there can be geographical restrictions on their operations. Make sure the lenders you contact can operate in your area.

2. Does your loan require PMI? And if yes, what does it cost?

    If they do charge PMI, this is not a true physician loan. Keep shopping to make sure there are no better options.

3. Is this a portfolio loan that will be serviced by your institution? Do you specialize in physician loans?

    As described in the chapter on physician loans, portfolio loans are usually issued using the bank's own funds and the bank will keep the loan and service it.

4. Do you offer fixed-rate loans? Do you offer ARMs?

Many banks that offer portfolio loans don't offer fixed-rate loans—they are all adjustable-rate loans of some kind.

5. Up to what loan amount will you finance 100% of the house price? Above that, how much down payment do you require? What credit score do you require?

Many lenders offering physician loans will do 100% financing up to around $750,000, and then require 5% down for $750,000 to $1-1.25 million, and larger down payments from there. Credit score requirements vary and you need to know you meet their specifications and will be offered their best terms.

6. What are your interest rate lock terms? Do you have the ability to float down the rate? How long can the rate be locked, and can you relock the rate? What is your lock fee and how is that paid?

Once you are ready to make an offer on a house, you will need to lock on an interest rate before your closing date. A standard lock period is 30 days. For most lenders, if the rate lock period expires before you close, they will likely charge an additional fee to relock. It might be an up-front fee. If you need a longer rate lock period, you may be charged a higher fee, a higher interest rate, or a higher closing cost once you get to the closing table. Some banks don't charge a fee for the lock.

7. Will you provide an itemized fee sheet for an example loan that breaks down the costs?

You don't want to waste your time applying with somebody and then find out they have a 1% origination fee. The low end on an origination fee is a flat $1,000, regardless of house size. Ask for an explanation of any fees or terms you don't understand on the fee sheet.

8. If I have been out of residency for less than 10 years, will you still finance 100% of the loan?

Some lenders restrict their best terms to attendings who have been out of residency for at least 10 years. Others will work with residents and students.

9. Do you charge points or offer buy-downs?

A point is 1% of the loan value that you can pay as an up-front fee to lower your interest rate for the life of the loan. Usually points will take too long to break even and are not worth paying for, however it's valuable to know if it's an option.

10. Is there a prepayment penalty on your loans?

Some lenders include a prepayment penalty in their loan terms. Look for a lender who offers competitive terms and no prepayment penalty.

11. What interest rate are you currently charging?

Specify a loan type with this question, such as a 15-year fixed or 30-year fixed, so you can compare across lenders. What you'll actually pay will be the rate you get when you request a lock, after you have an offer contract on a house. The answer you get now will be an estimate based on current market conditions.

12. Do you offer financing for noncitizens of the U.S.? If yes, do you accept a green card or a J-1 visa?

If you are not a U.S. citizen, your financing options may be more limited, but some lenders will accept J-1 visas or green cards.

You can download this interview questionnaire at DougCrouse.com

Getting Quotes From Lenders

You will receive a lot of information from mortgage lenders: current interest rates, locking information, an itemized fee sheet to help you estimate closing costs, and their required terms for the types of loans they offer.

The itemized fee sheet is an estimation of the fees you will pay at closing. Look for the origination fee, quoted interest rate, and other information to use for comparison against other lenders. Take note of any questions you want to ask to help you make a decision about which lender will be your best choice.

The itemized fee sheet is not a preapproval or a guarantee of terms, however the lender's fees should be accurate and provide information you can use to narrow your options to the lender you want to work with.

Once you have identified the type of loan you want and are preapproved, have a house under contract, and have requested a lock on the interest rate, you should get a *loan estimate* from your lender. This is a finalized version of the fee sheet. Your closing will be based on those final numbers, and you will use that information to determine how much cash you will need.

Remember, what the lender initially offers you doesn't have to be the final offer. You can negotiate, the same way you do for the purchase price of a new house. If there is a particular lender you want to work with but their interest rates or closing costs are higher than other quotes, give that lender a chance to match the other offers.

Guidance From the Lender on the Cost of a Home

You need your lender to help you understand the true cost of a home. If you are buying a home in an area with high homeowners association fees, you may need that information from your real estate agent.

Property tax rates, along with other local taxes, plus the cost of homeowners insurance (also called hazard insurance), vary significantly by state and area. For example, taxes in Texas are super expensive and in Missouri they are super cheap. Your lender will know how to estimate these for the area where you are shopping. A real estate agent may be able to ballpark these expenses but you need the numbers from your lender to be fully informed.

Understanding Closing Costs

Closing costs are the fees that make up the actual cost of borrowing money. When you buy a house, you've got to have the money in your pocket for the closing costs, down payment if you are doing one, and prepaids. So the closing costs are just one part of the cash you must bring to the table.

If you've ever heard someone talk about "rolling the closing costs into the loan," they were talking about a refinance. You can't do that on a purchase—those fees must be paid in cash at the closing.

Bigger House = Bigger Closing Costs

How much the closing costs are depends on the house purchase price, the lender's policies and fees, and the interest rate you get for your financing.

Some of the closing costs are charged as a percentage of the purchase price—so the bigger the house's price tag, the more closing costs you will pay.

Closing Costs Are Only Part of "Cash to Close"

Cash needed at closing will include closing costs and other expenses such as the *prepaid* items. This is money you can't borrow but must bring with you to the closing in the form of a certified check or by wiring funds.

Cash to close is made up of three things:

1. Closing costs, including origination fees and other related expenses—see list below

2. Prepaid expenses, which are the sum of the per diem interest based on the number of days to the end of the month from the closing date, plus one year's homeowners insurance premiums, and a portion of the property taxes to make an initial deposit into the escrow account

3. Down payment, if you are doing one

Closing Costs

Closing costs are fees paid one time to the lender at the closing of the loan. Not all lenders or title companies handle these exactly the same way (a few of these fees may be charged up front), but the following fees may be included:

- Origination fee

- Appraisal

- Title insurance

- Credit report fee

- Recording fee

- Rate lock fee (about half of lenders will add this to the closing costs and the other half will charge this fee up front)

- Other related loan processing fees

These fees are collected by the title company and disbursed to the appropriate people as part of the title company's service. The itemized fee sheet from your lender provides an estimate of these. Closing costs can often be negotiated.

Prepaids

Prepaids are expenses you must pay at the purchase of a house, and are made up of three things:

- Your first year of homeowners insurance premiums

- The escrow setup amount, which includes two or more months of taxes and insurance

- Prepaid (per diem) interest, for each day from closing to the end of the month (if you close on the 12th of the month, you'll owe the lender 18 days of interest to month's end)

Down Payment

Depending on your loan terms and your goals, this can be anywhere from 0% to 20% or more of the purchase price.

Debt-to-Income Ratio (DTI)

Your DTI (debt-to-income ratio) is very important in the qualification process. You can calculate your DTI on your own, so you have a general understanding of what the bank will be using.

List your monthly rent or mortgage payment, any child or alimony payments, auto loans and other products you have a monthly payment toward, student debt payments, and credit card payments (use the minimum payment). Add these items together.

Take your total gross salary and divide by 12. This is your monthly gross income. Divide the total of your monthly debts (X) by your monthly gross income (Y) to get your DTI ratio:

$$Monthly\ Housing + Monthly\ Debt\ Payments = X$$

$$Total\ Gross\ Salary\ /\ 12\ months = Y$$

$$Total\ Monthly\ Housing + Monthly\ Debt\ Payments\ /$$
$$Monthly\ Gross\ Salary = DTI$$

Multiply by 100 to get the percentage. Remember, the target ratio for physician mortgage loans is 45% or lower. The lower the number, the better chance you will qualify.

If you have a large amount of credit card debt or a vehicle loan and are still showing a $50,000-$60,000 resident's salary, you may run into issues with qualification. The best scenario is to pay down as much of your credit card debt and car loans as you can before you take on a mortgage. Not only will you put yourself in a better financial situation, but it will help increase your chances of qualifying for a loan.

You can download this DTI explanation as a PDF at DougCrouse.com

Preapproval for a Mortgage Loan: Why You Need It

Once you have identified the lender you want to work with and that lender has helped you identify the price range of house that you are comfortable purchasing, it's time to get preapproved. You will apply for a mortgage and the lender will review your information in depth and provide you with a letter stating how much they are willing to loan you.

There's a difference between being *prequalified* and being *preapproved* for a mortgage. Preapproval means your lender will do an in-depth review of your financials and name an amount of money they are willing to loan you. It means they have run your credit and looked at your background, your income, and your spouse's income, if that's applicable. Preapproval is essentially a mini-underwriting of your financial life.

They will state (in writing) something like, "Based on this information, if it doesn't change, we will give you a loan for up to this amount." Understand that this is not a guarantee, and you can still not be approved if something changes.

If they approve you for more than you want to borrow, you are not obligated to borrow the full amount.

You need to know how much you are preapproved to borrow before you start seriously hunting for a house. Then you can look for houses in your price range with the help of your agent and when you find the one you want, you can submit an offer with your financial paperwork in order.

Whether you are trying to apply for a physician loan or any other type of mortgage, getting a mortgage preapproval letter from a lender will show a seller you are a serious buyer.

Don't fall prey to mortgage brokers who advertise mortgage prequalification as it means absolutely nothing. Prequalification means that based on the information you have provided (that they have not verified) it appears you can obtain a home loan.

The Preapproval Process

Around three months or so before you want to purchase your house, go through the preapproval process with a potential lender. The reason you want to do this so far ahead is because your credit will be pulled, and you do not want too many inquiries to show up as you finalize your mortgage.

As you nail down your list of potential lenders, you need to work with one to start the preapproval process for the loan. You can use a lender for the preapproval process only—you are not obligated to use them for the loan, although approval guidelines and requirements can change from lender to lender. Most people go with the lender they are preapproved with.

Getting preapproved is an important step in the process of applying for a physician loan. You will quickly find out if there are any potential hiccups before you put an offer on the house. Often the first step is an online application. This application form will likely not say "physician loan" or "doctor loan" on it. A physician loan is a specialty version of a conventional loan.

HIPPOCRATIC HOUSE CHECKLIST

Paperwork for Preapproval

You will need to provide documentation of your income, including tax returns and pay stubs (unless you are a resident who has not yet started their new position), employment contract, bank statements, and your medical license if you are applying for a physician loan.

A typical request for documentation from the wage earner will include these (if you are not a business owner):

- ❑ W-2s for the last two years
- ❑ Tax returns for the last two years
- ❑ Two pay stubs
- ❑ Two months' worth of bank statements
- ❑ Most recent retirement account statement
- ❑ A copy of your medical license to verify you qualify for a physician loan

Collect the required paperwork into a file box that you keep in an accessible location. A common problem with physicians who are moving to a new area is they have packed all their paperwork in an inaccessible place. There is no substitute for your tax returns, so take the effort to collect these papers somewhere that remains accessible as you prepare to move.

Self-Employment Paperwork Requirements

If you are self-employed, your salary requirements will look different. You will have to submit two years' worth of income to show your salary is consistent and preferably has increased.

For self-employed physicians, the lender will average these two years together when calculating how much house you can afford.

Self-employed physicians will also have to show a strong credit profile and a low DTI ratio. Being self-employed doesn't automatically disqualify you from a loan. It only means you will have to show a consistent and stable work history.

Can Locums Doctors Get a Physician Mortgage?

Yes, you can still get a mortgage. The bad news is you are considered self-employed so you will go through a more rigorous process and have to provide more proof of your income. If you've been working as a locums physician for at least two years, don't let it stop you from trying to obtain a physician mortgage.

What Not to Do When Getting Preapproved

Applying for credit or closing an account will change your credit report and possibly critical things about your credit—your DTI ratio, for instance. You want to show a stable report, so don't make any changes to your credit accounts for several months before you apply for a loan, and don't make any *after* the application either, until after you close on the house.

- Don't close any accounts

- Don't open any accounts

- Don't make any big purchases (car, furniture)

- Don't be late with regular payments

You can continue to make typical monthly purchases as your credit report shows. Changing your debt-to-income ratio or letting your credit score take a hit from a credit inquiry will affect your standing with your lender. Don't assume they are not monitoring your credit, once you are preapproved.

In addition, there are other things you want to avoid at this point in the process beyond your spending. Pay attention to your regular bill payments and keep everything on time. Don't let something negative show up on your report. No matter how high your credit score is, it will be affected if you make a single payment late.

Don't let the amount of money the lender might say you can borrow go to your head. Stick to the monthly payment limit you determined before you approached any lenders. Don't forget that even if you aren't making student loan payments now, you will have to in the future. Your loan obligations won't disappear once you buy a house.

While getting preapproved with a lender doesn't mean you must do your financing with that lender, most people approach it that way. Make sure you've done your homework to choose a lender who has experience in the type of loan you want to utilize. If that's a physician loan, it pays to work with a lender who has years of experience in this kind of specialty financing.

HIPPOCRATIC HOUSE CHECKLIST

The Don't List for Preapproval

- ❑ Don't make any big purchases or take on new debt.
- ❑ Don't open or close any new credit accounts.
- ❑ Don't slip on making your current bill payments on time.
- ❑ Don't underestimate your student loan payments.
- ❑ Don't pick the wrong lender.

Grand Rounds by Dr. Tammy

One of Doug's previous clients planned to use a large nationwide bank for their physician loan, but two months later, the loan had not yet closed. When they finally got to the closing table, the closing costs were much higher than they expected. This should never happen with a good lender. You should have good estimates within a few dollars of your expected closing costs and a timeframe that is set up front. There are sometimes variables such as insurance costs or local fees that cause small changes in your closing costs, or delays caused by waiting on appraisals, but thousands of dollars or measuring time in months should *never* happen!

Chapter 5 Takeaways

 Choosing a lender is the first important step you should take in your homebuying process—before you choose a real estate agent and definitely before you start looking at houses.

 The right lender can save you money. Take the time to find a good one. Interest rates and origination fees are two things that can save you thousands.

 Prequalification and preapproval for a mortgage are not the same thing—they're like glancing at the table of contents compared to reading the whole book. What you need is pre-approval before you start shopping for a house, so you know what you can afford. Don't waste your time looking at houses you can't afford.

 While your lender may approve you for a loan at 45% debt-to-income ratio, you'll be a lot more comfortable with a ratio in the 30s. Don't go for the max—you'll find that limits your options now, and for sure later in life.

 The *itemized fee sheet* you can get from a lender is not guaranteed but is a quote of the expected costs and terms. Once you have a house under contract and have locked your interest rate, you will receive a *loan estimate*, which is a commitment from the lender. They must conduct the closing using those amounts—they are the final deal.

 Once you've been preapproved for a mortgage, understand that you need to put off any big purchases or new credit applications until after you've closed on your house. These things can change your credit report and your score (temporarily) enough to make your lender reconsider your approval. Don't assume they're not looking at your credit once the preapproval is complete.

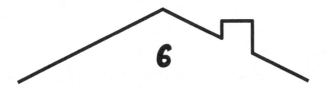

6

LOOKING AT REAL ESTATE AND WORKING WITH A REAL ESTATE AGENT

Where to Start?

As described in chapter 5, once you've decided you want to buy a house, your first step should be to shop for a lender. Lenders will know the specifics on interest rates, taxes, and other expenses that affect how much house you can afford.

While you are asking lenders for itemized fee sheets and interest rate information, ask them for real estate agent referrals. Lenders work with many agents regularly and can point you to experienced agents who understand the specific needs of physicians.

Before you engage an agent, however, you should spend a little time determining what you want and need in a house.

Define Your Priorities and Criteria in a House

Once you have a good idea of the house price range you want (with the help of your lender), your next step is prioritizing house features and location requirements. An obvious one is size of house and lot for your lifestyle, budget, and market. What fits your budget in one market may be half the size of what you can afford in a different market. Balance these aspects to find what works and makes you happy in the long run.

If you are married, you and your spouse should make your own lists of priorities for what you want in a house and neighborhood, and then compare.

Before you begin your search, understand that there are two houses out there vying for your interest: the one that meets your needs and the one that fulfills your dreams and desires.

In a perfect world, you would find a house that meets both, but in reality, you will have to make a choice. While it sounds like I am referring to the price of the house, that's not entirely what I mean.

For example, do you choose the three-bedroom house with room for your family to grow, or do you go with the house that has the massive backyard perfect for entertaining? Is it more important to have a bigger kitchen or the extra bedroom for guests?

These types of questions will come up, so make sure you know what is really important to you and what is more of a luxury that you could potentially do without.

When you start looking for a house, you will find homes that you fall in love with for different reasons. Having the list of features you want before you start looking can help keep you on track. Break it into two categories—needs and desires—and then prioritize the list. What do you absolutely need in your house and what can you live without?

You can start by looking at homes on sites like Redfin or Zillow. Don't rely on their estimates of home values as those tend to be incorrect, but the other property information is normally pretty accurate.

Take Your Time

Buying a house is a major decision so take your time and don't rush one of your biggest purchases in your lifetime. Buyers who rush into buying a house have a higher likelihood of making costly mistakes.

Build Your Team

Once you have determined how much house you can comfortably afford, make sure you have the right professionals around you. These include a financial advisor, a lender, and a real estate agent.

Your financial advisor can help you see the big picture. This person will help you devise a plan so you can pay off your loans and still enjoy the benefits of homeownership.

The lender's job is to present different options for financing that are available to you as a physician. They can provide calculations as to how different interest rates and types of loan products will affect your bottom line: the monthly payment. A lender may also be able to recommend a real estate agent, since they work with many. You want to find an agent who will represent you as the buyer.

A buyer's real estate agent will help you find the right house in your price range. That person can also help you negotiate to get the best price for the market and not overpay.

Finding and Working With an Agent

How do you find a real estate agent to represent you as the buyer? The best way is through referrals, so ask friends who they liked and who to avoid. If you're moving to a different town where you may not know anybody, ask colleagues you meet during your interview process.

One of the best places to find a good real estate agent is through your lender. A lender who provides loans for physicians will know good agents who work with physicians and understand their needs.

If you don't get a name you can work with from personal referrals, take a look at the names on signs in areas you are interested in buying. If you see the same name on multiple signs, give them a call. You know at the least that they are active and knowledgeable in the area.

Interview at least three agents and look for someone who has your interests as the buyer in mind. Ask questions and if you don't understand or aren't comfortable with the answers, move on. You need a good level of rapport with an agent, so look for someone who's easy to communicate with and who seems to understand where you're coming from. If they work with physicians regularly, that's a plus. Also check the Resources page in this book.

Real Estate Agent Versus Real Estate Broker

A real estate broker is somebody with a higher-level license that allows them to employ other agents. A broker can sell real estate as an agent, but they can also manage other real estate agents. An agent is only able to sell and must be employed under a broker's license. A broker may run a real estate agency or work solo as an agent. A broker can also work for another broker. Either a broker or an agent can provide the excellent service you are looking for.

Understanding Buyer's and Seller's Agents

A very common mistake is to buy a property through the agent who listed it. *You should never do that*—but it happens all the time. Real estate agents are paid by the seller, and typically their commission is 5-6%, which is split between the buyer's agent and the seller's agent. If you use the listing agent, that agent's going to get both sides of the commission. You may think that if you use them you'll get a better price because they can discount their fees—but they're not going to discount their fees. They just get paid more and now you've got somebody who can't represent both the seller and the buyer, so they become a transaction broker and basically, you just got a pencil pusher who's not really looking out for your best interest or the seller's best interest.

The agent's responsibility is to be your advocate. Your agent will work with the seller's agent to reach agreements in your best interest. A single agent cannot adequately represent the best interests of both the buyer and the seller at the same time; it's a clear conflict of interest. If you use a seller's agent, especially in a subdivision, that agent works for that builder day in and day out, while they're going to work for you once. You'll never get the kind of representation you would get with a buyer's agent.

Remember It's Your Money

As your advocate, the buyer's agent is there to make whatever offer you want. You want to benefit from their guidance and experience, but ultimately, it's your money. It's your house, so take in as much of their advice as you can and then use it however you want. Don't let your real estate agent decide everything for you. You should use them as your counsel.

You can do some of your own research too—jump on RealEstateAgent. com for valuations and Zillow.com for information about transactions. If you ask your real estate agent for comps of what is sold, you can jump on RealEstateAgent.com and see what a house sold for and what it looked like. You can't physically walk in it, but you can get an idea of the differences—say one had a kitchen from 1960 and another one had a $40,000 kitchen remodel. Although there are a lot of cookie-cutter houses, no two houses are exactly like each other.

Agent Interview: Questions to Ask a Real Estate Agent

Here are some questions to ask as you interview potential agents:

1. **How much business did you do last year—how many buyers, how many sellers, how many transactions?** Keep the current market conditions in mind when you ask this. If they sell fewer than 12 houses per year, they are likely not working full time. Keep looking for a full-time agent.

2. **How long have you been in the business?** You want someone with years of experience, not months.

3. **What price range were the houses you assisted in buying/selling?** You want an agent who knows the size and price range you are interested in.

4. **What neighborhoods have you worked in?** You want an agent who's familiar with the area where you want to buy.

5. **When are you available to show houses?** If your and your agent's schedules can't match up, you won't get very far. You want an agent who can be flexible and fit your schedule.

6. **Do you charge a transaction fee? If yes, how much and how should it be paid?** The real estate agent's transaction fee can be a "sleeper" fee that catches you off-guard when it shows up. It's the fee the agent has to pay to their broker. This fee can be around $400 and is in addition to the 3% commission the agent will make to handle the transaction for you. Ideally you want an agent who doesn't charge a fee. If they do and you like them and feel you can work with them, at least you know this fee is coming. Because both the buyer's agent and the seller's agent are paid by the seller, it doesn't save you any money to negotiate a lower commission in exchange for that fee.

7. **If I find a for-sale-by-owner house, what happens? Do I have to pay you even if I don't use your services in the transaction?**

8. **What kind of market are we in right now? What's the best strategy for getting the house we want in this market?** It's good to understand what the agent thinks is going on in the current market and how they think it should be handled. You can get a feel for this yourself from Zillow.com or through what agents tell you. You'll learn something about how they think and whether you are comfortable with them.

You can download this interview questionnaire at DougCrouse.com

A knowledgeable agent will have years of experience helping buyers and sellers. They will have a team of professionals they have used many times (lenders, home inspectors, movers, etc.) at your disposal. They will be able to provide you with comparative market analyses (CMAs, also known as "comps") that will help establish the value of the home you are interested in and assist in creating the best offer for you.

Don't settle on the first person you talk to. Wait until you find somebody who communicates in a manner you like, who is nice, who understands what you're looking for, and who isn't going to push you into just buying anything so they get paid.

Real estate agents get paid on commission, meaning they don't get paid unless you buy a house. So you don't want somebody who's just pushing you toward something even when it doesn't meet your criteria. You want somebody who will help you find the house that best fits your needs. They should ask what you need.

Contracting With an Agent

The first thing to know is if you sign a buyer's agent agreement, you're basically committing to that agent to represent you and you can't then go buy a house without paying them—unless you cover that circumstance specifically in the agreement. So if you sign a buyer's agency agreement and then find and fall in love with a for-sale-by-owner house, you or the seller will have to come up with the money to pay that agent. Sometimes a for-sale-by-owner seller does so because they don't want to pay a listing (seller's) agent, but they're fine paying a buyer's agent—but sometimes they won't.

Transaction Fee

You're also most likely agreeing to their transaction fee. Most agents will pass on to you the cost their agency charges them. It might be $395 or $495. Before signing with an agent, ask if their transaction fee is negotiable—because it *is* negotiable.

This real estate transaction fee is often a "gotcha" because it will be an extra fee at closing that has nothing to do with the loan, so it won't be on the itemized fee sheet from your lender. However it's a fee that you as the buyer agree to pay up-front to your real estate agent when you sign with them—if you read the fine print. It will show up at the closing table when the title company gets their list of fees the real estate agents require from you—because the seller is paying their commission. Each agent will likely make 3% of your house price from the seller—or $15,000 if it is a $500,000 house.

The contract you sign with an agent will not include the commission they will be paid when you buy a house, because you don't pay that fee—the seller does. That fee is predetermined by whatever the seller's willing to pay. As the buyer, the only part of the commission that's negotiable with you would be if you bought a for-sale-by-owner. You could put in your contract that, if you find a for-sale-by-owner, your buyer's agent's maximum compensation is whatever amount you want to specify. You would have to address that up front because once you sign, it's final.

Why to Consider Not Signing a Long-Term Contract With an Agent

A word of caution: beware of any agent that wants to push you to sign a buyer's contract with them for longer than 60 days. A better alternative is to sign a 30-day buyer's agency contract with the understanding that you will extend if the agent hasn't found you the perfect home but is doing a good job. That way you are not locked in with a lazy agent and have months wasted, waiting for the contract to expire.

Do your due diligence and find a real estate agent who has been in business 10-plus years. Hire an agent who is an expert in the area where you want to shop and who can provide referrals or examples of past deals they have closed.

Choosing an inferior agent will almost always leave you paying more since they aren't as skilled at negotiations. They might also be slow to communicate not only with the sellers but with you as well. Plus, you don't want them to waste your time looking at houses that really don't meet your criteria.

HIPPOCRATIC HOUSE CHECKLIST

Contracting With an Agent

- ❑ **Communicate to the agent that you want them to act as a buyer's agent.** You want to avoid working with a seller's agent without your own representation.

- ❑ **Identify the length of time for the initial contract.** No more than 30 days is a good place to start. Don't sign anything longer with a new agent, in case they don't work out.

- ❑ **Discuss transaction fees with the agent and ask if that is negotiable or can be waived.** These are negotiable fees and the agent will most likely be making 3% on the purchase price of the house you buy.

- ❑ **Discuss their compensation in the event that you find a for-sale-by-owner house and buy it without need of their services.** Be clear on who is responsible for paying them and how much it will be in that circumstance—it does not have to be the standard 3%. Some for-sale-by-owner sellers will pay the buyer's agent's commission and some will not.

The Process of Looking at Houses

You've found your agent. Now you need to start looking at houses. Your agent will set you up with email listings. They'll start off by sending you everything that meets your criteria, and you can choose to see those listings if you like them.

Then they'll take you through the property. If you like the property, walk through it again and look for things you hate. If you like the house, make sure you *really* like the house, and you don't just think the paint color is pretty, or you like the kitchen but everything else about it is awful.

If you can't live with an aspect of a house before you buy it, you won't be able to live with it after you buy it. You'll hate it and you'll want to sell it. There's a buyer for every house.

If you're looking at the worst house in the best neighborhood, it might mean some money needs to be put into it. But when you spend money on renovations, it will build equity by increasing the value of the home. If there's something you dislike about a house, consider whether you can fix that aspect, or if it's something you'd have to live with.

Location, Location, Location

This is a phrase we've all heard, but it's true. The location of a house is a big deal and is one of the main drivers of price stability and growth. Buying the worst house in a great neighborhood will always outperform the best house in a bad neighborhood, over time. Do not compromise on location; it isn't worth it.

Also ask your agent what kind of resale, growth, or rental potential exists in the area, keeping in mind that you can't time the market or really predict what's going to happen.

School Districts

Even if you don't plan on having kids, choosing a house within a good school district is always a wise decision. This is a common mistake, especially for those who don't have kids. So try to balance what you want with the potential resale value of the house. If you have kids, it's obviously important for them to attend quality schools, but even if you don't have kids, you want to choose a good school district because houses in those areas are more sellable and tend to hold their value better than similar homes in weaker school districts.

This is part of how you "make your money on the purchase," meaning you buy with selling in mind.

You need to buy with selling in mind.

What kind of schools you are looking at will depend on the age of your children and whether you want private or public schools. Neighborhoods with the best public schools tend to be more expensive. If your children are young, try to consider schools as they grow older. Choose an area that can be good for everyone on a long-term basis, as much as possible. People sometimes feel forced to move because of location alone; take the time to consider your long-term plans and needs so this doesn't happen to you.

Local Crime Rates, Roads and Railroad Tracks, and Flood Zones

Check the local crime rates when evaluating your new house. When you have narrowed it down to a house you really like, drive by it at different times of the day to check traffic flow and traffic noise. Take notice if the home is in a flood area or is near a railroad.

Convenience to Work and Play

Consider how valuable your commute time is, based on your expected work and on-call patterns. Do you have to be able to get to the hospital within 20-30 minutes? Surgeons, ER, and any trauma-related specialties will be glad they chose a house close to work. The time you save could be significant.

Workplace proximity is a huge consideration for your work-life balance. Consider the budget in that balance because closer can be more expensive. But it's undeniable that too much time spent commuting adds stress and other expenses to your life. If both spouses work, this can get complicated. Knowing the area will make this aspect of the decision easier as you will be familiar with traffic patterns and alternative transportation options.

While the commute to work is important, the locations of other services and amenities are often overlooked. Pretend you are driving to the grocery store or other errands you frequently make to see if the house you like is in a good location.

There are several factors to consider about the neighborhood you choose to buy in. If you are new to the area, consider renting for six months or a year to find out where in town you want to live. As you find your way around a new area, you will get a feel for where you really want to be.

Neighborhood Look and Feel

You don't want to choose a house and find out in two weeks that you hate the neighborhood. Some things cannot be seen on a drive-through; a wrong decision can impact your life and your finances in far-reaching ways.

Is the house next to an apartment complex that doesn't have enough parking? They'll be parking in front of your house on nights and weekends. Is the street a convenient cut-off route to avoid busy streets? You won't feel safe letting your kids play outside. Before you buy, visit the area at different times of day and night to see what's going on.

One Time When It's Good to Be Smaller

Take a good look at the size of houses in the neighborhood and especially on the block with the one you like. A common mistake for physicians is to end up with the biggest house on the block. Those are the hardest to sell. You're actually better off buying a middle of the road or the smallest house in a nicer neighborhood.

If houses in the neighborhood are selling for $400,000 and there's one that's selling for $300,000, take a good look at that one. Even if it needs renovation or updating, that additional expense is a relatively small amount of money spent that you'll be able to recover on the sale.

People who want to pay $300,000 are looking in the $300,000 neighborhood, and then they find that same size house in the $400,000 neighborhood, and they say, "Ooh. I would live there." If you have a $400,000 house in a $300,000 neighborhood, people who are looking for $400,000 houses are looking in $400,000 neighborhoods. So, that's going to be more difficult to sell.

Look at Market Predictions in Your Area

Research the market predictions in your area. See how the local housing market fared in the recession and research what the projected growth might be in the future. Also understand that the unexpected can change everything.

If neighborhoods in your chosen area are declining or have poor quality or shrinking school districts, it's probably not wise to buy. However, if housing prices are steadily rising or even beating the average growth nationwide, it might be a good time to buy.

Other Things to Consider in Your Search Process

People move and have to sell their houses for many reasons. Most of them don't matter to you as a potential buyer, unless they are moving because they no longer like the area due to recent changes.

When you find a house you are seriously considering, ask a few more questions to make sure this could be a good purchase for you.

- **Ask your real estate agent to find out how long the seller has owned the house.** It could be a red flag that the seller bought the house a year and a half ago.

- **It's very useful information to know what the seller paid for the house.** These are both matters of public record so your agent can get this information.

- **Also ask your agent to find out why the seller is selling, if there is an opportunity.** Note that in a hot market, you likely won't get the opportunity to ask questions like that. But in a slower market, it's worth asking. There are certain things a real estate agent and the seller are required to disclose about a property, and this isn't one of them. But if they are honest, it can be useful information. You may find out there's a new mall going in across the street that will impact traffic significantly. Often, the reason is something like a job change, divorce, retirement, or downsizing.

HIPPOCRATIC HOUSE CHECKLIST

House Hunting

❑ **Define your priorities and criteria for a house.** List size, number of bedrooms, features, lot size, garage details, and anything else that's important to you (big utility room or pantry, for instance).

❑ **Communicate the price range you want to your agent, along with your other priorities and criteria.**

❑ **Discuss location, location, location with your agent.** School districts, proximity to work, shopping, other community amenities. Identify subdivisions or other areas where you want to live.

- Identify school districts

- Identify homeowners association restrictions you do or don't want (these end up having big impacts on your life)—can or cannot park an RV or other item on the property, for instance—and request your agent to obtain the HOA CC&Rs (covenants, conditions, and restrictions) for specific subdivisions.

Grand Rounds by Dr. Tammy

Having the right real estate agent can be just as important as having the right lender. Both can help you save thousands of dollars and many headaches. Most experienced real estate agents can spot potentially hazardous or costly details in a house when walking through with you. They should be aware of market trends and be able to see the history of a given house to help you negotiate. Your lender can help you find an experienced agent who works with professionals in your desired neighborhoods.

Chapter 6 Takeaways

 Your lender is in a perfect position to refer you to an experienced real estate agent who can make finding your house easier. They work with dozens of professionals and know which ones know their business and which ones specialize in working with physicians.

 Choosing the right house can be an emotional decision, but it's also the biggest or one of the biggest investments you will ever make. Keep an "exit strategy" in mind when you shop for a house—what characteristics will make your house easy to sell, when that time comes? Keep those aspects with universal appeal in mind when you choose, so you don't end up with something that you want but nobody else wants.

 Even if you don't have children, start with the best school districts in your search for a good neighborhood. Houses in good school districts hold their value better and are in greater demand.

 Understand that many aspects of the real estate transaction are negotiable, even if they aren't stated that way. This includes the agreement with your real estate agent, the fees you pay, and the contingencies you specify.

MAKING AN OFFER

Understanding the Market and the Seller

Are you in a buyers' market or a sellers' market? Understanding this drives many aspects of the process and negotiation. If you're in a buyers' market, you're in the driver's seat and can make an offer based on what you want to pay. And you can expect that the seller will consider a below-market offer. There's no hurry and you might get a great deal.

If you're in a sellers' market, you're competing. If it's a hot sellers' market, you can expect to be beat out almost every time you make an offer. Somebody's going to come in and outbid you. In that circumstance, some real estate agents will direct you to make a high or even an exorbitant offer. There are problems with that—if you get the high bid that's great, but if the appraisal doesn't come in as high as your offer, you have an issue. You can only borrow an amount based on the lesser of the purchase price or the appraised value. So paying way over the market value won't help because when the appraisal comes in short, then you'll either have to make up the difference out of your own pocket or the deal will fall apart.

How Do You Know What Kind of Market You're In?

If you have been looking at all, it will probably be obvious. As you work with your agent, you'll find out how long houses are on the market before they sell.

If they're on the market for a few days to weeks, it's most likely a sellers' market. If they are on the market for 90-plus days, that's probably what's called an *even* market. And if they're on the market for longer than four months, that's usually considered a buyer's market. You can avoid hot markets by shopping in the "off-season" from late fall into early spring. Fewer people are looking at that time of year and inventory tends to be higher.

Determining an Offer Price

So you found a property and you want to make an offer on it. Your agent will submit the offer, most likely using an online document-signing service. Tell your agent how much you want to make an offer for or ask your agent to help you determine the best offer to make. Remember it's your money and will be your house—so benefit from your agent's expertise in what's a fair offer for the market conditions and ask for their guidance, but make your own decision. You can research prices on websites like RealEstateAgent.com and Zillow. Zillow is good for transaction history but RealEstateAgent.com may be a better source for valuations.

Based on the market conditions, there are a few more pieces of information your agent can provide that will help you decide what's a fair price.

Comparisons

Ask your agent to run the comparable properties (or "comps"), which is a list of similar properties that have sold recently in the same general area. Another type of comparable report you can request is a list of all the properties that have sold in the same subdivision over the past 12 months. If the subdivision is small, include five or six comparable houses within a certain radius around that subdivision. This will give you an idea of typical appreciation in the area.

As for what "recently" means, if you're in a really hot market, it's about three months. If you're in a lukewarm market, you can go back six months. If you're in a cold market, you could go back as far as a year or whatever it takes to find some sales.

If all three-bedroom, two-bath houses with a three-car garage in the area are going for $400,000, it isn't a good idea to make an offer for $200,000.

Most likely it won't get accepted. But does that mean you have to offer the asking price? No. You could offer $395,000 or $375,000. Maybe another one has brand-new everything and the one you are offering on has old carpet and dingy paint or something else that's unappealing.

You want to look at properties that are in similar condition to the one you're buying, if possible. You decide on a price with your agent, taking advantage of your agent's guidance. Understand that your offer price is not based on the listing price, no matter what it is.

Work to view the process objectively and keep looking for other houses, even after you put in the offer. If you become emotionally attached to one house, you may pay too much for it and regret it later, or else bid so aggressively that the appraisal doesn't agree and the deal falls apart anyway.

Hot Market Strategies

If you are shopping in a hot market, you will be in competition with other buyers and you'll likely be offering the asking price or higher. You might also be outbid regularly for desirable properties. If it's an even (moderate) or slower market, you've got more time and more clout—that is, you may be able to offer something less than the asking price and get it. The market also affects how you set up the contract. How you do contingencies may be different.

If you are in a hot market and you need to find a house soon, you may need to also find a "plan B" house. Sometimes people regret doing this, but if it's a high likelihood that you will be outbid, you shouldn't necessarily stop shopping for a house just because you found one you like or you have an offer out on one. Until you have an accepted offer and appraisal back, it's smart to continue to look.

There is a chance you will find another house you like better than the one you're under contract for, and you may have buyer's remorse if you go with the first one anyway. There are also legal ramifications, depending on what you do: you could be sued for non-performance if you renege on the first contract because you had to have the second house. You would also likely lose your earnest money.

Bidding Wars in Hot Markets

You'd like to avoid buying in a hot market but it may be a fact of life. In a hot seller's market (this is very relevant on the East and West Coasts, and in many other areas post-COVID), you can do what's called an *escalator clause*. This is a way to circumvent a lot of the hassle of a bidding war and avoid paying more than you have to for a house.

An escalator clause basically says that you will pay X number of dollars more than your initial offer up to a specified maximum. For example, say you want to buy a house for $500,000 but you don't know what anybody else has offered (and it's typical that you won't know), so you offer $475,000 but agree to pay an amount (say $1,000 or $2,000) higher than any other offer that's made, as long as the final amount doesn't exceed a limit you specify. It's a sort of bidding process with a cap. That way, you only pay more than your initial offer if someone else's offer beats yours.

This type of clause removes much of the back-and-forth interactions that can happen in a bidding war, which you don't have time for. An escalator clause allows you to make an offer and then sit back and wait to see if it is accepted.

In the absence of an escalator clause, how multiple bids are handled is up to the real estate agent representing the seller. They can disclose as much as the seller allows them to. If I was a listing agent and I had multiple offers, I would go back to the low offer with the high offer and try and get my low offer to surpass my high offer, knowing that if I don't get that, I would just take the high offer.

So sometimes the low offer gets to counter. The agent goes back to the low offer to negotiate and then take that offer back to the better offer and see if they want to beat that. So they essentially are creating an escalation clause without actually using one. The reason an agent can get away with that is the seller was given too much time to decide. Or if it's a house's first day on the market, sometimes 10 offers may come in on one house.

In the last five years with online listings, some real estate agents will intentionally underprice a house in an online listing to create a bidding war. People need to understand that's what's happening. They see a house online and think, *This is a great deal! I want this house. It's priced at $300,000.* Some agents will do this, knowing they'll get multiple offers to create the bidding war. Like going to an auction, people pay more to outbid the next guy, versus paying closer to what they would have paid for it if it was priced correctly. So the $500,000 house ends up selling for $540,000—and then, good luck if it appraises.

Earnest Money and Contract Negotiations

The earnest money is basically a pledge that you intend to move forward with the transaction. And if anything goes awry this money is not automatically returned.

> Pay just enough earnest money for the
> seller to take you seriously.

Many real estate agents will say the best amount to pay is in the range of 1-2% of the price of the house—but that is negotiable and there is no hard-and-fast rule. If the transaction does fall through, it becomes a legal issue as to who gets that money. It's not a given that you will get that money back. You might have to go to court for it.

A good rule of thumb on the earnest money is to keep it small enough that you won't mind too much if you lose it. It's possible to put up $500 on a $500,000 sale—just enough so the seller will take you seriously.

Before you write the check, discuss with your agent how your earnest money will be handled, and under what conditions you could lose it. Typically this happens if you simply change your mind even after all contingencies are met, or something unforeseen happens that you didn't cover with a contingency.

At closing, the earnest money is typically applied to your closing costs or prepaids and if any is left over, you will get the remainder back at closing— "cash back at closing."

Escrow Account

Earnest money is placed in escrow when you make an offer on a house. The real estate agent will arrange for an escrow account—an account set up by a third party to hold the earnest money from the day you make the offer to the date of closing.

A different type of escrow account is set up by the loan processing company to hold the funds from your monthly mortgage payments and from those funds, pay property and other taxes and homeowners insurance. The "prepaids" portion of your cash required at closing will go toward the initial funding of that escrow account, as required by the mortgage company.

The Contract

The contract is the agreement the buyer and seller negotiate to cover the purchase price, down payment amount, and any contingencies to be included. It also includes several details that can have a big impact on the outcome, such as how long your offer is good (when the seller has to reply by) and the closing date. House inspection contingencies and finance contingencies both have the potential to make a deal fall through. Make sure you have the information you need from your lender and communicate with your agent so these details can all work to your advantage as much as possible.

As long as it's not a hot market, there's no rush in putting the offer contract together. So until you've got it drawn up and presented, you've got as much time as you want to take. However, if it's a hot seller's market, then while you're drawing your offer up, somebody else may have already presented theirs and given the seller four hours to decide. So again, the kind of market you are in affects the entire transaction.

There Is No Such Thing as a Standard Contract

Ideally, ask your real estate agent for a blank copy of the offer contract well in advance of making an offer so you can read it. Especially read the fill-in-the-blank parts because that's where the dates are—closing date versus date of possession, for instance. Those should be the same date and time. That is, you want to take possession on the closing date and not one or two days later.

And yes, read the boring fine print—sometimes those details become quite important if the negotiations or one of the contingencies take the deal on a detour during the process. Some of that is negotiable and some may not be, but knowing it will help you make the best decisions and avoid problems.

Offer Time Limit

One big mistake many people make is giving the seller too long to decide. You can specify this in the contract, and sooner is better, from the buyer's point of view. Ask for an answer the same day, ideally, and no more than 24 hours. Don't worry about disturbing someone's weekend or evening—you can ask for a decision in four hours, by 10 p.m. on Friday night, if you want to. Because if you make an offer on Friday and ask for an answer by noon on Monday, the seller has the whole weekend to go shop with every other person who's looked at the house to say, "I've got this offer of $500,000. Do you want to make your offer now and compete with them?" This is more important in a hot market than a slower one, but the principle is the same.

Giving the seller too much time to make a decision on your offer puts them in the driver's seat. You want to be in the driver's seat, so push for an early decision.

There's More to the Contract Than Price

In order to put together a good contract, you need information from both your lender and your real estate agent. Each of them will have requirements that you put in the contract as contingencies that must be met, or the contract is void. These are for your protection.

Some contingencies are standard and some may apply specifically to the circumstances or the house. Many people don't discuss with their agent what contingencies should go into the offer contract before they are drawing it up, but they should. Earnest money—how it's handled and how much—and a host of other critical details like a previous sale contingency (not applicable if this is your first house, of course), home inspection, and other inspections should all be discussed with your agent, and you both should agree on how they will be handled. Contingencies are discussed in more detail in the next section.

You should also ask your agent to find out if there are any other offers pending on the house before you write yours up. If it's a hot market and there are several competing offers, you may need to make your offer as competitive as possible for it to be considered. However if you're not competing with another offer, you'll want to start with what you want to offer. But if you know for sure there's at least one other offer on it (some agents may not be honest about this, but if they're being honest and you know you're competing), then you want to put your best foot forward on your first offer because otherwise you might get passed over on a house you really love. You may also want to utilize an escalator clause.

An offer to buy a house is a legally binding contract and once the seller accepts it, you can't change it. So whatever you need for a closing date, the amount for earnest money, and any other items—such as if you're asking them to leave an item with the house, remove something from the property, or repair issues found in the inspection (termites, for example)—all that has to be decided up front as you're making your offer.

Request Possession at Closing

Ask your agent to set up the contract for possession at closing and include both time and date. You need to request that up front or you may end up in a situation where you're allowing the seller five days to get moved out. It's one more detail to check before you sign the contract.

Those details need to be communicated between the buyer and the real estate agent. Every deal is different. There's no set standard that the buyer will get possession at closing, but you can request it.

What often will happen without this request is, for example, the closing will take place on May 15 and you don't take possession of the house until May 17. Or it may be a matter of hours—the closing takes place at 10 a.m. and the contract says you take possession at 5 p.m. You might show up right after the closing and the seller hasn't moved out yet because they've got until 5 p.m.

When you have that gap—when you've closed but don't have possession—you're taking a risk that somebody else owns your house during that time, even though it's yours. You'll do a walk-through before closing, but there are opportunities to damage the house between the time you did the walk-through and when you actually own it.

In order to take possession at closing, the title company has to get those final documents out to get approval for funding the loan, and most title companies want to wait until that has happened before handing over the keys. Some lenders are not as efficient as others in getting those documents transferred. The title company sends them to the lender, and sometimes it might be hours before some lenders get an approval out, but it's possible to do it in 15 minutes, if your lender is customer service oriented.

The Closing Date

The closing date is always specified in the contract, and this is often negotiated between buyer and seller and can depend on contingencies. Sometimes someone will say, "I need to close on this house in three weeks." That could be an issue, and it depends on the appraiser. If the appraisal can't be done in time, then three weeks is probably not realistic. You as the buyer also need to provide updated information to the lender—more recent pay stubs and bank statements, for example. Four to six weeks is much more reasonable, and trying to rush it can lead to problems.

When the Seller Becomes a Renter

Sometimes the seller requests to stay in the house for a period of time, often several weeks after it's sold, and rent from you. Your real estate agent can negotiate this for you. Obviously you won't take possession at closing in that case, however you may want to work out a damage deposit agreement just like any other rental. Your lender usually doesn't want to see this kind of arrangement, but it happens frequently and it can be to the benefit of both buyer and seller.

The expectation of the lender is you will move into and occupy the house within 30 days of closing. The reason for this is when you are in the house it is less likely to suffer a loss due to theft or damage, such as a water damage, where no one was present to remedy the problem.

Contingencies and What They Mean for You

Contingencies are steps that must take place before the contract price can be paid. They are always some kind of "out" for the buyer, reasons why the contract can be canceled. There are some standard contingencies you, as the buyer, want to have included in the contract. The contract will go through if all of the contingencies are met.

These basic contingencies are present in the majority of contracts:

- House inspection: the house must pass an inspection by a professional house inspector.

- Mortgage financing: the buyer (you) must be able to obtain financing.

- House appraisal: a house appraisal is required by the lender and that appraisal must come in at or above the agreed-upon purchase price, or else the lender will not loan the amount you request.

- Sale of an existing house: if this is not your first house purchase, you may need to have sold your existing house by a certain date as part of the conditions for your loan approval and therefore it must be included in the contract for your new house.

Here are more details on some of these contingencies.

Home Inspection

Most first-time house buyers and probably 80% of repeat house buyers will have the house inspected and make their offer contingent on their approval of a professional home inspection report. Most physicians will want to do a whole-house inspection, however not everyone does it.

If you don't get a house inspection, you should ask questions like when was the roof replaced and how many layers of shingles does it have? What other work has been done to the house in the last five years? Your real estate agent can ask those questions for you.

If you get a house inspection, the inspector will probably tell you those things.

There's a sense of required honesty from the seller, if you ask them questions like these. They can be held liable if they outright lie. There's a seller's disclosure clause in the contract, most of the time, and if their statements are not accurate, they can be held liable for deceiving information. You would have to sue them for damages to get that money, though, and it may not be worth it.

A house inspection will give you peace of mind and it can protect you from some unpleasant and costly surprises, so you want to hire a good inspector who will look out for your interests. The older the house, the more important an inspection is, although even new houses should probably be inspected. However if the new house has a home warranty, this may not be necessary.

The Buyer Hires the House Inspector

As the buyer, you should choose the house inspector. You can find one through a personal recommendation or ask your agent or your lender for recommendations. You should always accompany your inspector during their walk-through to discuss anything potentially wrong with the house that the seller failed to disclose.

A house inspection will cost you between $400 and $800 depending on what sort of tests you're doing. Typically you as the buyer will pay the home inspector directly, completely separately from the loan transaction or purchase, although it can be included in the closing costs in some cases.

Once you've agreed to a price with the seller, you can't typically negotiate repairs or compensation on any issues without having a qualified house inspector doing an inspection. If I look at a house myself and say, "I see the bricks are falling off," they're not obligated to fix that. But if I had a home inspector go out and inspect it, typically that would open it back up for negotiations.

Keep in mind on a house inspection that whenever you go back to the seller after the house inspection and make new requests, that basically unlocks the contract because you're saying you're not willing to accept it as is. If the seller says they're not doing a thing, then that opens the opportunity for them to walk and cancel the contract.

At that point you just lost out on the house you wanted. Sometimes people get hung up on $500 worth of stuff in a $500,000 house. That's 1%. It's silly to lose a house you really want over principle on a small amount like that because of other money you've already tied up in it.

No house is perfect. You need to consider all the factors and recognize that even a brand-new house can have problems.

There are additional inspections you can have done and add them as contingencies, for several other potential issues.

Termites

In any area with even a remote possibility of having termites, get a termite inspection. A termite inspection is cheap and the typical contract will have wording something like this: "If termites are found, the sellers will at their expense pay to eradicate them." So that's a cheap investment because termite inspections are sometimes free on purchases and at most, probably $75. That could potentially save you anywhere from $400 to $1,500 in a termite treatment, and if termites are found, the sellers have already agreed up front to pay for it.

Radon

Radon inspections have become pretty relevant in recent years. I've bought a few houses with radon pumps. They're not a big deal but people can be freaked out by them. So if that might bother you, it's not nearly as cheap as a termite inspection but not as expensive as a whole-house inspection.

Sewer

It's important to be familiar with state regulations regarding house construction and hookups to utilities. For instance in the state of Colorado, the homeowner is responsible for the sewer pipe from the house to the middle of the street. If that's the case in your state, you should also do a sewer inspection. I recommend all my clients get a sewer inspection because that is a $7,000 fix or more.

Say you didn't pay $400 or $800 for the house inspection and now you have a $7,000 bill to fix the sewer pipe that you didn't know was broken. But if you had found it before you bought the house, you could've asked the sellers to fix it, or you could've split the difference and had a $3,500 bill instead of a $7,000 bill. So, you definitely want to know the condition of the house and make sure you are comfortable buying the house in that condition.

An inspector might tell you to get something checked out by another professional. For example, if the AC isn't working, they might say you need an AC expert to come look at it. That's going to be an additional cost, but it's probably worth the money spent to find out you'd have to replace the whole AC unit.

Attend the Inspection

Make a point of attending the inspection and walk around with the inspector, watch, and listen. "Oh look. This light switch doesn't work."

You say, "Okay. Is that a big fix?"

"Well not really. It's probably a couple of dollars." The inspector isn't likely to give you a hard-and-fast quote on how much it will cost to fix something, but they will know if it's a $10 fix or a $10,000 fix.

They will not remember your house after they leave because they inspect many houses a day. So you need to be there with them to take notes and ask questions.

The house inspection is an overview of problem areas. It's up to the buyer to understand the report. The buyer must find someone who specializes in any identified problem areas for more in-depth inspections, if needed.

This is a time to pick and choose your battles. Some things you should ask the seller to fix, but you don't necessarily want the seller to fix everything. They may not choose quality appliances if something needs to be replaced. It is much better to get cash up front and choose the appliance for yourself.

If you are buying your first property, you don't know what a broken foundation looks like. Do you know that the pipes work? A house inspection is not a guarantee that the house will not have any problems ever, but the house inspector comes in and says, "Oh look. That furnace is 12 years old." A furnace typically will last for 13 to 20 years. You want to know about this so you can either ask the seller to remedy the problem, ask them to lower the price, or ask them to split the difference. For many people, it doesn't matter if it's your first or your 30th purchase—you don't skip the home inspection.

Mortgage Financing

A finance contingency is a definite requirement to cover the possibility that the market changes unexpectedly and you can't get the interest rate you need. At a minimum that should be a statement like "This offer is contingent on my getting a loan at 4.5% or less." Then if you can't get a loan except at 10% and that's not acceptable to you, you can back out of the contract using the mortgage contingency.

You will have decided what type of loan, whether you want a fixed-rate or variable-rate loan, and what loan period you want during your preapproval process. You were preapproved for up to a certain loan amount based on some assumptions about the current market, including the interest rate. You want to include a contingency in your contract that states those assumptions and limits how much they can change before you would be unable to obtain affordable financing for the purchase.

Appraisal

No one with "skin" in the transaction should choose the appraiser to satisfy the appraisal contingency before the closing can happen—not the buyer, the seller, the lender, or the real estate agent. The appraiser is selected by an independent third party through Appraisal Management Company (AMC). You will likely be paying the appraiser separately and at the time of the work.

Because of the 2008 housing crash, new regulations were put in place to create a degree of separation between the appraiser and everyone else. This was done because people were influencing appraisers and manipulating numbers to the point of making deals work that shouldn't have. Now, there are big fines for trying to influence an appraiser.

On the contract, make sure you check the house appraisal contingency box. The appraisal must come in at or above the offer price because the lender will not loan you more money than the house is worth. So if the appraisal comes in below the offer price, without that contingency to give you an out, you have to make up the difference.

If that happens (appraisal is lower than the agreed-upon sale price) you have two options:

1. Come up with cash for the difference on the loan.
2. Ask the seller to reduce the price to match the appraisal.

Without that contingency, if you can't make either of those options work, the deal could fall through.

You do have the right to ask the seller to reduce the price to the appraisal price, but they can say no and walk away.

Setting the Closing Date

Set the closing date a reasonable amount of time into the future. What is reasonable depends on the state of the market—just like determining the offer price and just like finding a moving company. Once the contract is signed with a closing date specified, it can be a problem to change it. So think carefully when setting it in the first place.

If interest rates are low and refinances are surging as a result, the same appraisers, title companies, and closing agents are busy with refinances as well as purchase transactions. A glut of refinances will create a backlog that slows down everything, so be aware of that impact on your closing date and choose a doable date.

If you can set up and make an offer to close in a time frame that's still acceptable to the seller, four to six weeks is a lot better than trying to do it in three to four. There are restrictions on some paperwork that the buyer has to sign days before closing. Lenders must have certain documents to the buyer, and the buyer has to have a certain amount of time to review them.

Four Weeks

As a general rule, don't schedule a closing less than four weeks from the contract signing. If there's a house sale contingency in the contract, six weeks is a more realistic minimum, especially if money from an escrow account is needed for the closing. You and the lender will be going back and forth with updated paperwork and things to read and sign. If you try to close in under four weeks, it will be stressful for you as the buyer and you will likely regret it.

The biggest issue with a short close is the unrealistic expectation for when an appraisal can be completed. Ideally the appraisal due date and termination on the contract should be only a week less than the close date.

HIPPOCRATIC HOUSE CHECKLIST

What to Include in the Offer Contract

Your agent will put together the contract and that's what you are hiring them for. Ideally you have seen a blank one before you find the house you want to offer on. Discussing the contingencies that should be included in the offer is also useful to have on the table before the contract is set up.

Here is a list of details to include in an offer contract:

❑ Offer price

❑ Earnest money

- Amount you will offer

- Who will hold it (who will set up the escrow account)

❑ Contingencies (discuss these in advance with your agent if possible)

- Home inspection

- Termite inspection

- Sale of previous home to be completed by a specific date

- Items requested by buyer that seller leaves with the house

- Items requested by buyer that seller must remove

- Appraisal termination date

- Finance contingency (may be called mortgage contingency)

❑ Closing date

❑ Closing/title company

❑ Closing location

❑ Request for possession at time of closing or a date following closing

An Accepted Offer

Making an offer is one thing; having a seller accept it is another. Almost always you'll get a counteroffer with at least one thing changed. Sometimes it's just a matter of dates to accommodate the seller. Sometimes they want different earnest money. Sometimes they want more money. Sometimes they want all of it and it might be that you asked for an heirloom light fixture to stay that they said wasn't staying.

So you'll get a counteroffer, which the seller will sign. The seller doesn't sign your offer—they only sign the counteroffer, which basically says everything in the original contract stands except these items and then the buyer and seller both sign just the counteroffer.

Once you get an accepted offer, typically the next step will be to provide the contract to your lender and start the inspection process, if you're going to inspect the house. Any other contingencies requiring inspection or other scheduled services are also set in motion.

Inspect Before the Appraisal

Ideally you want to inspect the house before the lender orders the appraisal. Because once you order the appraisal, that money is spent and gone, and if the house contract falls through because you find things wrong with it during the inspection, you're out the cost of an inspection *and* the cost of an appraisal. The decision could have been made before the appraisal ever happened.

If time allows, get the inspection done first, then green-light the lender to move forward with the appraisal.

After or simultaneously with the appraisal, you'll probably be working with your lender to provide updated pay stubs and bank statements, and maybe an employment contract if it's a new job.

Title work is also ordered about that time. The title work will basically show that the seller owns the property with just the encumbrances of a mortgage. The title work and resulting title insurance is to make sure some other contractor didn't come in and finish a rec room and never got paid, or something else that could result in a lien against the property.

If you are buying a newly constructed house, the lender and/or title company orders a plot survey to make sure the house is on the correct lot and the garage doesn't sit on the property line or some other violation of the easements.

Your Loan Interest Rate: Deciding to Lock or Wait

Deciding when to lock the interest rate is a strategic decision and it is not in the contract. With most lenders, you can't lock a rate until you have a house under contract. Whether you lock the rate right after the contract is signed or wait until closer to your closing date is your choice. Ask your lender for guidance on when to do this, taking your closing date into account.

Once you lock a rate, that's the rate you'll close at, whether the market goes up or down. It's kind of like a marriage—it's for better or for worse. If the interest rate goes down, you've already chosen to lock; if the interest rate goes up, you're protected.

It's also kind of like buying stocks. You'll never catch the bottom and you'll probably never catch the top either, so you can't expect that. Decide if it's good and go for it.

If you choose not to lock your rate immediately, stay in contact with your lender on a regular basis. Even a small rate reduction can make a difference—so if it dips, you can lock on that because it will be better than you had before. Even an eighth of a percent on a big loan might make $50 to $60 per month difference in the payment.

Start Preparing for the Move

It's easy to forget about the practicalities of moving in the excitement of buying a house and trying to fit in all the related tasks. But now is the time to start the ball rolling for your move.

First are the details of leaving your current location. First-time homebuyers will typically be giving notice on a rental. Decide how much overlap you will need between when you take possession of your house and when you leave the old place and give notice according to your lease. Research moving companies or get recommendations from friends and colleagues and schedule that service. Think about giving notice for any utility accounts in your old place that need to be shut off.

At the other end, you need to set up all the utilities for your new house. Ask your real estate agent to obtain the names of utility companies that service your new house and contact them to give them your information to transfer the accounts, including the dates you want that to happen. You don't want to get there in freezing cold or a heatwave and find the power, gas, or water off.

Grand Rounds by Dr. Tammy

Making the offer and waiting for the response can be so exciting! It's like waiting to find out if you got into the residency program of your choice. Most of the time, deals sail through with no major hiccups. Sometimes things don't work out as you hoped, but like in life, I think things happen for a reason. Doug has told me about a few cases where the appraisal didn't come in as high as the offer. This can actually work to your advantage and be a reason to renegotiate a lower price. Be ready to pivot if your first choice doesn't go as planned.

Chapter 7 Takeaways

 How you make an offer, the price you offer, and other aspects of negotiating the contract depend on whether it's a buyers' or a sellers' market. Be sure you understand the current environment and discuss this with your agent so you understand how your agent intends to negotiate for you.

 Read the offer contract thoroughly before signing it, and understand everything in it.

Contingencies protect you against common issues, so make sure you understand what they are for and how they will affect the process and closing.

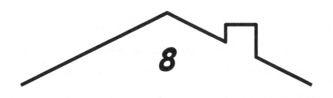

CLOSING

Preparation for Closing

When an offer contract is signed, a series of steps are put into motion that culminate with the closing, funding, and handing you the keys. These steps take time and closings are typically scheduled 30 days or more from the date of contract signing.

Paperwork Updates

Soon after or simultaneously with the appraisal, you'll probably work with your lender to provide updated pay stubs and bank statements, and maybe an employment contract if you are getting a new job.

Your lender may not verify your assets at the preapproval stage, but money for a down payment will definitely need to be verified prior to closing. That's why you need the two months' bank statements or the source of funds to show that you have the money for the down payment.

When You Are Not a First-Time Homebuyer

If you are not a first-time homebuyer, sometimes down payment funds are coming from another house sale. In that case, the lender will want a copy of the closing disclosure for that sale to see what the proceeds were. Also if some of the money is coming from an escrow account, those can be delayed. Don't assume when you're selling a house that you'll have all the money sitting there to pay next year's taxes and insurance on the new house, or that the money will be credited to the payoff. That's not typically the case.

So if you're waiting on an escrow refund, your previous lender needs to know where to send it. If they don't know, it may be sent to your old house, where it will have to go through the postal system to be forwarded to you. You may be waiting another two weeks to get your money. A previous house sale contingency usually requires more time before closing on a new house because of these details—six weeks may barely be enough time.

People will sometimes overestimate how much money they'll have for the down payment and this can be problematic. If the lender approves you with the assumption that you've got $47,000 and you actually end up with $42,000, that won't work. The closing costs and prepaids must be paid in cash too, and if they are more than anticipated, that can cause a shortfall. Or if the loan amount is different (higher) than you were approved on, this can happen. Be careful that you can verify whatever amount you say you have.

Title Work

The title work for the title insurance policy is also ordered during this time. The title work is the title research and documentation to show that the seller owns the property with only the encumbrances of a mortgage. The reason you need title insurance is to make sure some other contractor didn't do work on the house previously and never got paid. Title insurance protects the new buyer. It's the title company declaring, "If there are other encumbrances and we didn't find them, that's on us."

If you have a question, ask the title company. People who have worked in the industry for 20 years sometimes don't understand title insurance and what it covers, so don't expect that you will. You need to ask questions and get the title company to explain what they are covering in plain English so you understand. Don't feel that you should know it or pretend that you do—just ask.

Survey for New Construction

If you are buying a brand-new built house, you'll probably have to get a plot survey too. The lender takes care of the survey with the title company. It's an added expense specifically for new construction. It's a survey to make sure the house sits on the correct lot and the garage doesn't sit on the property line. Because the house is brand-new and has never had a survey, both the title and lender will require one.

Locking on the Interest Rate

You have to lock on the interest rate before closing, possibly by as much as a week. So if you weren't locked soon after signing the contract, this needs to happen so the loan can be finalized and the required paperwork completed prior to closing.

Down Payment and Cash at Closing

The cash you need to bring to the closing can be handled one of two ways—either a cashier's check or a wire. People sometimes think they can write a $50,000 personal check. Most title companies won't accept that. You need to know your final closing amount before the day of closing so you can stop at the bank and get a cashier's check.

Wires are common but can be very risky. You can get hacked and end up wiring the funds to the wrong place. If that happens, the money is gone. You cannot get it back.

If you have to do a wire, confirm twice that you have the correct wiring instructions from both the lender and the title company, and you may want to call to confirm with the institution before sending it. My preference is always a cashier's check if possible.

Understanding Prepaids

Prepaids are made up of three things: your first year of homeowners insurance premiums; the escrow account setup amount, which includes two-plus months of taxes and insurance; and per diem interest, which is calculated per day from the closing date to the end of that month. The total will depend on when during the month your closing is scheduled. For example, if you close on the

12th of the month, you'll owe the lender 18 days of interest to get to the end of the month.

Your first mortgage payment after closing is always going to be a month after the first day of the month that follows your closing. So if you closed on April 9, your first payment is due on June 1. The per diem interest is for the remaining days of April.

When you make your June 1 payment, the interest portion of that payment is for May's interest. That's why the per diem interest is collected only for April—from April 9 to April 30. The earlier in the month you close, the more per diem interest you'll pay. You also have a longer grace period between the day of closing and your first payment, because if you close on April 9, you'll have 51 days until your first payment. If you close April 30, you've only got 31 days. Many people prefer to close near the end of the month to minimize the amount of prepaid interest they will have to pay at closing.

You can ask your lender for an estimate of the prepaids, and those amounts will be known except for the per diem interest. Once the closing date is set and your interest rate is locked, they can give you real numbers on the interest per day from the day of closing to the end of the month.

Your lender's itemized fee sheet may include an estimate of one day's interest based on the quoted interest rate. They can explain the per diem interest and show you fees for closing at the beginning and the end of the month. Some lenders will show 15 days of prepaid interest in their fee sheet as a middle-ground option, and can say the worst case is double this and the best case is none of it, depending on your closing date.

The homeowners insurance is not always paid at closing; you may have the option to pay it separately, in advance.

The escrow account setup amount is typically a reserve of two months' worth of the annual property tax bill and homeowners insurance premiums.

For property taxes, the seller must pay at closing the portion of the year's taxes up to the date they sell the house. However, you may need to pay more than two months' worth of property taxes in order to have the required cushion for the escrow account, so ask your lender for that estimate.

Closing

It's a good idea to schedule closing closer to the beginning of the week than the end of the week. You do not want a late closing on Friday, because what if something happens? Your bank is closed. They won't open until Monday and you were planning on moving in on the weekend, and now you can't.

Whether the closing is being handled by a title company or an attorney, talk to whoever is performing the closing several days in advance and ask them, "Can I bring a cashier's check? What identification do you want me to bring with me when I come to the closing? What do I need to do?" You must have final numbers on the cash needed to close so you can bring a cashier's check in the correct amount to the closing.

Final Walk-Through

Many agents will ask if you want to do a walk-through before closing. It's not a bad idea to do that right before you go to the closing table. Have the agent meet you at the house and do a quick walk-through just to make sure everything you agreed on in the contract happened. You can make sure the sellers actually moved out, took all their furniture, and didn't leave you a bunch of stuff to have to deal with when you move in. It's a good time to check for the unexpected, like if the sellers took light fixtures down or took the refrigerator and it was supposed to stay. It's a lot harder to get that resolved after you've closed and they've got their money. This is the reason you ask for a walk-through and it's something your realtor will negotiate with the listing agent to resolve.

Possession

The date and time you take possession will be specified in the contract. You can ask your agent to *request possession at closing* so there is no gap in time between when you close on the house and when you have possession.

Note that if you are renting the house to the seller for a period of time, protecting your property becomes very difficult because you will not take possession until the rental period is over. If possible, get a damage deposit from the seller to cover any damages you may incur.

Funding

Typically the transfer of ownership takes place when you've signed and the money is paid. But the recording of the transaction is often delayed. The title company may not complete the recording until the next day or even the end of the week.

What *finalizes* ownership is funding. When the money changes hands, that doesn't necessarily mean the public is aware of the event. So whenever the change of ownership gets recorded is when it's a public record, but the time of recording isn't when a property changes hands. Whatever the contract says is when it changes hands. Typically, it's when the loan funds, and that's whenever the title company's and the lender's bonds are released to the seller.

Behind-the-Scenes Details

In preparation for the closing, the lender will send funds to the title company the night before. Right after the buyer and the seller are done signing, the title company has to send a few documents, called backdoor closers, to see that those documents were signed. Then the title company will get an email saying they're okay to fund. Those documents include these:

1. Closing disclosure
2. The note
3. The deed of trust or mortgage

At that point, the title company can hand you the keys. They have approval to transfer funds to the seller and record the transaction.

The title company will act as the bank in the sense that they're the distributor of funds. In a few states, the money transfer is handled through an attorney's office instead of a title company. But more states use title companies to handle the closing, and the title company acts as a go-between. They collect the closing costs, prepaids, and down payment, coordinate the funding with the lender, and transfer the funds to the appropriate parties:

- Purchasing funds from the lender (and buyer if doing a down payment) to the seller

- Origination and other lending fees from the buyer to the lender

- Fees from the buyer to the real estate agent, the appraiser, and anyone else they are working with

- Prepaids to the lending institution's loan servicer

- Commissions from the seller to the buyer's and seller's agents

- Closing, recording, title insurance, and notary fees to the title company or their agents

If money is being wired for the closing, that is handled through the title company. The title company also handles the recording of the transaction with the county courthouse.

HIPPOCRATIC HOUSE CHECKLIST

Closing Costs and Prepaids

Here is a checklist of things you can expect to pay for at the closing:

- ☐ Closing costs
    - ☐ Appraisal
    - ☐ Title report and title insurance fees
    - ☐ Closing fee
    - ☐ Recording fees
    - ☐ Underwriting fees
    - ☐ Any other loan processing fees
    - ☐ Points (if you are paying them)
- ☐ Prepaids
    - ☐ Per diem interest on the loan from closing day to the end of that month
    - ☐ First year of homeowners insurance
    - ☐ Escrow account setup amount for the initial deposit (this could include at least two months' worth of taxes and the homeowners insurance premium)
- ☐ Down payment

These fees and how they are paid varies by state. They are also affected by the terms you negotiated for the sale and your loan, and by the title company's practices.

Things That Can Go Wrong

There may be surprise fees or the seller is not ready to give up possession. If you're building a house, delays could happen. Here are some things to watch out for as you prepare for the closing.

Final Verifications

There are a number of things that can cause a delay, but often it's something in the final verifications. Right before closing, banks will re-verify employment. It is done within the last 10 days of closing but recently, because of COVID-19, some lenders have started confirming at 10 days and again just before closing to make sure nothing has changed. Also be aware that banks will recheck your credit around this same timeframe to insure no new credit has been opened. For this reason, as much as you want to go out and buy blinds, etc., to be ready when you move in, you should *never* open a new account to do this or any other unusual purchase. Ideally, don't make any new charges that would increase your balances over what they were at the time of application.

Don't Disturb Your Credit

Many people have a misconception about the preapproval process, assuming that once the lender tells them their loan is approved, they can go do anything they want and it doesn't matter—no one will see. And that's not true. Your lender will check credit again before closing.

From several weeks before the preapproval process until after the closing, don't do anything that might affect your credit without your loan officer's permission. Don't charge anything except the normal gas and groceries you typically would. Don't miss a payment and definitely don't buy anything new.

If any credit inquiries appear on your record, you'll have to explain them in detail. Don't go shopping for a car and let a car lender pull your credit because that might affect the underwriter's decision. The underwriter might decide, if you're already at a 44% debt-to-income ratio, that as soon as you buy that new car, you really can't afford this house.

Construction Delays

If you are buying a new built house, any delays to final modifications to the house or finish work could delay the closing.

Who Still Gets Paid If the Deal Falls Through?

Only a few of the players will get paid whether the deal goes through or not. These are any house inspectors and the appraiser. Both of these are typically separate transactions and they are paid up front, at the time of service, and not at the closing.

If the deal falls through, the lender doesn't get to loan the money, the real estate agent gets no commission, and none of the insurance policies will be sold. The title work done by the title company will not be compensated for either, in the case of a failed deal.

HIPPOCRATIC HOUSE CHECKLIST

Contract to Close and Preparing to Move

A signed offer contract sets in motion the efforts of a whole team of people who have to work together to meet the contingencies, coordinate paperwork and funds, and finalize the transaction. At the same time, you've got to think about preparing to move.

It's a bit simpler for first-time homebuyers because you don't have to sell your old house before you can close on the new one. Buy you may still have to give notice on your current lease, determine what work has to be done before you move into the new house, plan the move, and make sure the power, gas, and water will be on when you get there.

❑ Coordinate updated proof of income and assets with your lender (pay stubs, bank statements).

❑ Read and sign any pre-closing paperwork your lender needs in a timely manner.

❑ Decide when to lock the interest rate on your loan and stay in contact with your lender until you do.

❑ Plan the logistics of moving your possessions and shop for a moving company or rental truck, etc.

- ❏ Give notice on your current lease.
- ❏ Verify your cash to close amount and that you have the funds for closing.
- ❏ Contact the title company and confirm how you need to provide the funds—preferably a certified or cashier's check rather than wiring funds.
- ❏ Shop for homeowner's insurance, select a company, and set it up with a starting date when you take possession.
- ❏ Ask your real estate agent to obtain a list of utility companies that service the house from the seller and confirm the date you will take occupancy and how utilities will transfer and not be shut off.
- ❏ Contact all utilities and provide billing information and the transfer date.

Grand Rounds by Dr. Tammy

Before I met Doug, I bought a small house and didn't shop for homeowners insurance. The real estate agent said they had a policy that could just be rolled into the contract and I signed for it at closing. A couple years later, I was talking about it with a friend who was appalled at what I was paying in insurance for my very modest little home. I can't stress enough that working with reputable real estate agents and lenders and doing some due diligence can save you so much time, money, and irritation.

Chapter 8 Takeaways

 There are many moving parts and necessary steps to prepare for a closing. Because of this, it's rare to see a closing scheduled for less than 30 days after a contract is signed. Sometimes a contingency in the contract causes the closing date to be pushed out much further than 30 days.

 The deal isn't done until the closing happens as planned, all paperwork is signed, and you are handed the keys. Up to that point, there's a chance something can happen to cause the deal to fall through. The large majority of deals go through as planned but be aware it's not guaranteed.

Your real estate agent and your lender can be instrumental during the preparation for closing in making things go smoothly, so rely on them and ask questions as needed.

The final cash (in the form of a certified or cashier's check) you will be required to bring at closing cannot be determined until the closing date is set. Specifically, the prepaids are affected by when in the month your closing date happens. The closer to the end of the month your date is, the smaller that amount of prepaid cash will be. Ask your lender for an estimate of the cost per day that will need to be calculated, so you can be prepared.

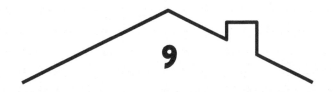

THE HOUSING INDUSTRY FROM START TO FINISH

The process of obtaining a mortgage and purchasing a house requires the services of several supporting industries. Laws at the federal, state, and sometimes local level affect how real estate properties are financed, bought, and sold. In addition, lender requirements drive some of the supporting services, including the appraisal and insurance industries.

Regulations at the state level can vary significantly and make house buying, selling, and financing look different in each state. Local taxes and property values also have an impact on how business is conducted.

From the buyer's perspective, what these people do in the process and how they are paid may not be transparent. Understanding how they are paid and by whom is helpful as you navigate the system.

Here's a list of the behind-the-scenes people involved in the house-buying process:

1. Lenders
2. Real estate agents and/or real estate brokers
3. Title companies
4. Escrow companies
5. Notaries
6. Insurance companies: homeowners and private mortgage
7. Appraisers
8. Home inspectors
9. Attorneys

Lenders

You can obtain a mortgage loan from a mortgage loan officer at a bank or credit union, or from a mortgage broker. There are also *loan servicing companies* that handle the payments and may also handle the escrow account.

Mortgage Loan Officers or Mortgage Brokers

You may work with a mortgage loan officer or mortgage banker, who is affiliated with a financial institution, or you may work with a mortgage broker, who can obtain financing from and sell it to a variety of other banks.

Because physician loans are portfolio loans, meaning they are specialty products offered by a financial institution using that institution's money, most physicians will work with a mortgage banker.

How the lender gets paid depends on whether they are doing a secondary market loan (all conventional loans) or a portfolio loan. If they doing a secondary market loan, they are a correspondent or a broker to the bank they sell the loan to. They are paid a set percentage of the loan, which they use to generate a new loan for a different lender.

Lenders are also paid through origination fees for the underwriting or for processing tax service-type fees. For portfolio loans, since they are not selling the loan, lenders get paid by servicing the loan. They borrow money at one rate and loan it out at a different rate.

The loan officer who works for the lender is paid a set percentage just like a real estate agent, and that percentage is determined between the loan officer and the bank (lender).

In summary, lenders are paid only when they loan money. Their payment is usually in the form of an origination fee plus the interest they charge you. If they sell the loan, they will obviously make money on that sale.

You will see the fees they charge in two places, typically. First, when you are shopping for a lender, you can request an itemized fee sheet, which will list the lender's origination fee and a quoted interest rate. You'll see the finalized fees they will charge for your loan and closing in the loan estimate, once the contract is signed and closing date is set.

Real Estate Agents and/or Real Estate Brokers

You may work with a real estate agent or a real estate broker. The broker can either handle real estate transactions for themselves or they can own a real estate agency and license other agents to handle them. The difference between an agent and a broker is the type of license they hold. An agent always must work for a broker, but the broker can sell houses or represent buyers like an agent if they wish. Only a broker can own a real estate agency.

It's actually a violation of law for the real estate agent to receive money from anybody other than their broker. When you have a contract with an agent, in reality you have a contract with their employing broker. That broker pays your agent.

Brokers can also provide a broker price opinion (BPO), which allows you to ask a broker what they think a house would be worth. That's typically done by the seller and costs a small amount of money, such as $35-$50.

The real estate agent's broker is paid by the seller, whether they are representing the buyer or the seller. The buyer's agent and the seller's agent split the commission, usually 5% or 6% of the sale price, which varies by state and location. That commission is also negotiable, between the seller and the agent.

As the buyer, you have no control over how much either the buyer's or the seller's agent is paid. However, when you contract with an agent, you are contracting with them to represent your best interests and negotiate on your behalf.

There's a misconception about real estate agents that all they ever do is show you houses. There's a lot more to it than that. They set up and negotiate the contract on the house. They are the go-between with the seller's agent and work to coordinate the home inspection and the appraisal and the title company and many steps that you may not see. There are a lot of dates and deadlines to be met.

As the buyer, you won't see the real estate agent's commission amount. However, agents may also charge a transaction fee, often $395 or $495, and when you are contracting with a buyer's agent, you should ask about this fee.

This fee may not show up anywhere except in the contract you sign with your buyer's agent and then at the closing as an extra fee—this one can be a "gotcha" or surprise fee at the closing if you don't know to ask about it.

When the seller pays the agent's commission, the money goes to that agent's broker (from the title company or attorney handling the closing). If the deal falls through, the agent or broker will not get paid.

Title Company

In many states, the title company acts as the bank in the sense that they're the distributor of funds. They also pay any other bills that were sent to the closing table. They collect all the money from the buyer and the lender, and they distribute it to the seller, the real estate agent, the insurance agent, the lender for prepaid interest, and anyone else who is due money.

In just a few states, the money transfer is handled through an attorney's office instead of a title company.

The title company gets paid for the title insurance, which has two parts. One part of the payment is for the policy and the other is for doing the research. They sometimes break those into two fees, but they are both labeled title insurance.

The title company also gets paid a closing fee for their services as the distributor of funds. That closing fee could be anywhere from $250 to $500, depending on your area and the title company.

As the buyer, you can choose the title company you want to work with. Most lenders will not refer one. Many people buying a house go with whoever their real estate agent recommends. Typically a real estate agent has a relationship with one title company and that's who they use. In certain states, there's very little difference between title companies in terms of cost. In other states, you might save $300-$500 on the title insurance and associated fees if you shop for a title company.

In around 50% of transactions, the buyer's agent will close at one title company and the seller's agent will close at another title company. You may not see the seller at all at the closing.

As the buyer, you will see the title company's fees in two places: an estimate in the itemized fee sheet and the confirmed fees in the *loan estimate*. The loan estimate will be used at closing and states the guaranteed numbers all parties will use to complete the closing. Your lender will coordinate with the agents on both sides and the title companies to include all fees in the loan estimate they provide to you.

If the deal falls through, even at the closing, the title company will not get paid.

Escrow Companies

An escrow company functions as a neutral third party to hold funds and documents for real estate transactions. The earnest money you pay when you sign a contracted offer on a house will usually be placed in escrow. Loan servicing companies use a different type of escrow account to hold the tax and insurance portions of your monthly mortgage payments until they are needed to pay the property tax and insurance bills.

Escrow fees are paid at the closing and are included in the loan estimate.

Because physician loans are portfolio loans—owned by the bank that loaned you the money—the bank may have escrow and loan servicing operations in-house, and there may be no separate escrow company or fees. However for conventional loans, the escrow company could be a separate entity.

Notaries

A notary signing agent acts as a witness during the closing and walks you through the signing process. Their fee is included in the closing costs.

Insurance Companies and Agents

Insurance in this case means homeowners insurance, not title insurance. Homeowners insurance is required by lenders to protect the house that is the collateral for their loan to the new homeowner.

The buyer shops for and selects the company they want to use, then pays for homeowners insurance. You will pay for insurance at the closing and continue to pay it in each monthly mortgage payment.

Appraisers

The appraiser is selected by an independent third party through AMC (Appraisal Management Company). The appraiser doesn't work for anyone else involved in the house-buying process. You may pay the appraiser separately and at the time of the work, or sometimes the appraisal fee is included in the closing costs, in which case the title company pays them. Your lender and/or your real estate agent will coordinate the appraisal.

House Inspectors

House inspectors are paid by the buyer directly, usually at the time of service. You choose the house inspector and can also choose other types of inspections including termite, sewer, electrical, and anything else you feel needs to be done. Your real estate agent will know inspectors for many of these and you can also get recommendations from friends and colleagues.

Survey Companies

Surveys are only required on new construction, and their fees are paid by the title company and will be included in your closing costs. The lender will request the survey be done.

Attorneys

Certain states require that an attorney be involved in the closing. The attorney may provide some of the paperwork services that could be provided by the title company. Attorney states include Oklahoma, Texas, and several East Coast states. The attorney's fees are included in the closing costs just like the title company's.

Grand Rounds by Dr. Tammy

You should always find a lender who specializes in doctor loans. Working at a bank that offers them isn't the same as working with a loan officer who does 10, 20, or 30 of them a month.

Chapter 9 Takeaways

 Many professionals are involved behind the scenes to make a real estate transaction happen.

 Understanding how those people are paid and who they work for can help you understand where they fit in the process and how that affects you.

 It's important to hire a neutral third party for the appraisal. There is a national organization that supplies this service called AMC (Appraisal Management Company).

 For home inspectors, you want to get a personal recommendation from someone you trust, if possible, and make sure that inspector has no ties to the seller. You want them to represent your best interests because you are paying them.

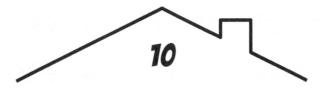

MOVING IN, COMMON MISTAKES, AND THINGS TO KNOW FOR YOUR NEXT HOUSE

When it comes to readying the new house for you to move in, the moving process, and any upgrades or repairs you are doing, you need to plan ahead. Renovations and repairs in particular will take longer than you think.

If you're buying a house that's not brand-new, think of it like buying a 10-year-old car. You better expect something's going to need work or replacement. Cars are expensive to fix, and houses are just as expensive. Plan on an air conditioner, furnace, or a water heater needing to be replaced. Consider yourself lucky if it's the water heater, as those aren't usually big-ticket items.

As you approach your closing date, start planning for the move by planning to have the utilities transferred to you.

Set up Transfer of Utilities and Clarify the Transfer Date With the Seller

People often don't think about all the contact information they will need for utilities—trash, electric, natural gas, water. You don't want to show up to your house on a Saturday when you're moving in and discover you don't have running water and can't call the water company until Monday.

As you plan your move, you may not think about the shut-offs at your old house (if you have one), and making sure everything's turned on in the new house. If it's in the middle of the winter, people don't think about keeping the heat on. Typically, the gas company wouldn't turn off gas in the middle of winter, but they're not obligated to keep it on so you need to reach out ahead of time and make sure they know you're taking over ownership at X date and give them your information for billing.

The usual practice is for the seller to leave the gas and electric on for a few days after the closing. But don't assume that will happen—communicate with the seller when you will take over the accounts.

The Moving Process

Moving takes much longer than people plan for and often costs more than they think it will.

Find a moving company as far in advance as possible, if you need one. Renting a truck to do it yourself requires similar planning plus the added detail of picking up the truck, driving it to your new house, and returning the truck. When you get bids for truck rentals, be aware that some states (California is one) require levels of liability insurance that can make the rental fee double or more the cost it would be in a neighboring state. It may be worth a detour and extra driving, so check prices in neighboring states as well.

Sometimes the timing of events requires renting a storage unit as an interim spot for some of your possessions. This is common when people are selling a house because a sparely furnished house will show better than a cluttered one. If you rent an apartment or house, you may have a storage unit already and your move will need to collect possessions from two places.

If you own the house you are moving from and will be selling it, timing is important. You don't want to completely pack up the house you're selling while you're still trying to sell it because it shows nicer if it's full—but at the same time, you don't want to have two days to get everything packed up and moved into the next house.

Home Warranties

Because you're buying something you're not familiar with—that is, you may not know what's already been replaced—you've got to be prepared for anything. If this concerns you, a home warranty may be a good idea for the first year, whether your home is new or not. That way you have some level of protection for the unknown.

After you've lived with the furnace and air conditioner and everything else for a year, you'll know if you want to extend the warranty. If anything seems like it's on its last leg, you may want to renew the home warranty. Or if everything looks good and you expect it to last another 10 years, then don't waste time or money renewing the warranty again. New construction will often include a one-year warranty.

If you are comfortable with home repairs, a home warranty may not be worth the money, but for most busy physicians, it may be worth it. Whether or not a home warranty is worth it also depends on how you prefer to buy insurance, in terms of deductibles. For instance, if you prefer to go with a higher-risk $2,500 deductible on your homeowners insurance policy, you probably won't get a lot of value out of a home warranty. If you prefer policies with a $500 deductible, you'll be more likely to benefit from the warranty.

Your real estate agent has relationships with third-party home warranty providers and can set the warranty up for you.

Read the Fine Print

Read the fine print if you're buying a home warranty. Know what you're getting because they may have deductibles or limitations on who provides services. For instance, many have limitations on any type of geothermal, such as a ground-source heat pump furnace and air conditioner—they're probably not covered because they're so expensive. Also, it's likely that high-end appliances will not be covered.

If you are doing any initial renovation such as paint and flooring or anything more involved than that, you'll want to consider doing as much of the renovation as possible before you move in. Begin by finding reputable vendors to do the work. Each vendor must come out to the property and give you a bid. Vendors may be reluctant to overlap bid appointments with other vendors, which can create problems. When you interview vendors, first check reviews and references.

Choose which company to use and schedule when they will come to the house and do the work. Make sure there is a set deadline for when the project will be finished, and insist the vendors behave professionally with each other. These steps will help ensure your projects get completed in a timely manner.

Common Mistakes in the House–Buying Process

It's not surprising there are opportunities for mistakes from beginning to end of the house-buying process. Here are some of the common ones and how to avoid them.

1. Shopping Before You Know What You Can Afford

It can be heartbreaking to go look at $700,000 houses and then find out you can't afford more than $550,000 because taxes are much higher than you anticipated. Figure out your comfort level and your budget first, and then talk to a lender. Talking with lenders should be your first step after you've determined the monthly payment you can handle. The lender can tell you the price range of house your monthly payment can buy, taking local taxes and other expenses into account.

2. Hiring a Real Estate Agent Who's Not an Expert

Do your due diligence and find a real estate agent who has been in business 10-plus years and preferably sells houses full time. Hire an agent who is an expert in the area and who can provide referrals or examples of past deals they have closed.

Choosing an inferior real estate agent will almost always leave you paying more, since they aren't as skilled at negotiations. They might be slow to communicate not only with the sellers but with you as well. Plus, you don't want them to waste your time looking at houses that really don't meet your criteria.

An expert in the area will be able to run comparative market analysis for the house you are interested in buying. They'll also be able to help nail down a price range that will help you get a house with most of the things on your wish list.

3. Not Taking All Expenses and Debt Into Account

Just because your lender excludes your student debt in your physician loan doesn't mean you shouldn't factor in your current and future payments. This is especially true if you are still in training with low payments and are in an IBR (income-based repayment) program.

It's important to think about future increases in your wages and expenses to make sure you can afford the house in the long term (five-plus years out), even if you do not intend to be in that house in five years.

The market can turn at any time (just like the stock market), so don't get caught having to stay in a house that you stretched your budget to get into. Instead, plan and crunch the numbers as much as possible before making one of the biggest purchases of your life.

4. Being in a Rush

A common problem I see, especially with residents, is they are in such a hurry to move and take care of things that their important papers are packed somewhere and they can't get them—and there's no substitute for your tax returns when you're getting preapproved for a mortgage. Take the time to put your important papers in an accessible spot so it won't end up in the back of a U-Haul that you can't access.

5. Not Knowing the True Cost of a House Before You Make an Offer

Before you make an offer, make sure you know the true cost of the house you are considering. The most common add-on fee is the homeowners association fee, and these can vary from none to several hundred dollars per year to over a $1,000 per month (in Hawaii, for example). Asking about HOA fees should be a standard question for any house in a subdivision or development. Condominiums can have very high HOA fees too.

In addition to HOA fees, ask if the community has any city-imposed special fees. In Las Vegas, these are referred to as SIDs (special improvement district) and LIDs (local improvement district) fees. In California, these fees are commonly referred to as Mello-Roos.

You can think of these fees as another form of property tax on your new house. The fee is placed on the house when the city installs services to what was an undeveloped portion of land that the developer builds on. A few examples of what the fees could represent are for sewer plumbing, roads, streetlights, or fire hydrants. When it's a brand-new house, the developer can choose to pay back the loan and increase the cost of the house to cover, or they could let the fees stay with each house and have the new homeowner pay it back over the next 10 or 20 years (an average length of time need to pay off these fees).

If you aren't buying a new house, some if not all of this fee will be paid down, but you still need to be aware that it might exist. While the fees vary by area, they commonly range between $50-$300 per month. They can be as high as $500 per month and amortized over 40 years. That is a potential $200,000-plus responsibility on top of the mortgage, HOA, property tax, and normal fixed expenses like gas and electric.

Ask your real estate agent if these kinds of fees could apply where you are shopping, and if yes, ask them to confirm the status of any such fees for any house you consider. Knowing how much they are and how long you would have to pay them should factor into your affordability evaluation for any house.

6. Buying the Biggest House on the Block

It's cool to be that family with the big house, but keep in mind the perceived value when you go to sell. You won't get a great price when yours is the biggest one on the block—the smallest house on the block gets that prize. Look for the middle range or smaller house on the block to get a boost in home value from the bigger ones next door.

7. Making an Emotional Decision Instead of a Rational Decision

Maybe you fall in love with a house because of its view, a wonderful kitchen, or some other aspect, but it doesn't really suit your needs. Perhaps the location isn't right or it's more than you want to spend. This tends to happen particularly if you begin shopping for a house before you know what you can afford and find that the houses within your price range don't live up to what you hoped.

Remember a house is also an investment and your return will come when you sell it—so thinking about its appeal to a potential seller as you shop for it can help you make more rational decisions. You want to avoid the white elephants and keep the location appeal as a primary consideration.

8. Focusing Too Much on Interest Rates

It's easy to focus too much on the interest rate when you are setting up your mortgage financing, thinking you have to get the best, lowest rate possible.

You *do* want the lowest rate you can find—and it's worth interviewing several lenders to compare the rates they offer because there can be significant differences that could save you hundreds per month. But don't pay points to lower the interest rate without a careful risk-benefit calculation. Most of the time it's not worth the money because it takes too long to break even.

For instance, if you can get a 3.5% rate with no points but it was going to cost you two points to get 3.0%, you have to weigh the cost and benefit of paying $10,000 (for example, on a $500,000 house), when it's going to lower your monthly payment by $100. It would take a long time to break even—in this case, divide 10,000 by 100 to get the number of payments you have to make to break even (100). You won't start saving money on that lower interest rate until after you've made 100 monthly payments—eight years and four months. That's too long—you might not even still own that house by then. You would have been better off investing that money in a mutual fund.

A related problem is thinking this house is your forever house when statistically, chances are good you won't be. If you're buying your first house, you may not be there more than five or six years. People sometimes assume that because they're buying a house they fell in love with, they're going to be there forever. If you're buying your second or subsequent house after your first house, 10 years is a long time. You don't know what will happen. Try to look at it pragmatically and ask yourself if you'll be there long enough to save more than it cost you. In the housing industry, a "forever home" is one you live in for 10 years.

My personal rule is don't buy points unless the break-even date is no more than 42 months (three and a half years) out. The same thought process and calculation applies to a refinance.

> If it takes more than 42 months (three and a half years) to reach the break-even point, don't pay for points or do a refinance. It may cost you more than you will save.

Also, don't expect to lock your interest rate on the absolute lowest rate for your loan. Watch the market, work with your lender, and simply choose a time to lock and—just like the stock market—be happy with getting a competitive rate. Don't expect to play the market because you can't see the future. When it looks good and is in the ballpark of your affordability range, make the decision and go with it.

9. Not Requesting Taking Possession at Closing

The timing of possession and closing can be confusing. Don't assume that they will hand you the keys at closing—you must specifically ask for it. This is important because you don't want the seller to still have possession of your house after you've closed. Because you do your final walk-through at closing, if you don't take possession right away, there is a period of time in which the seller may still be living in your house and has an opportunity to damage it or not follow through with aspects of the contract. This could be items to be left on the property or taken when they move out. Especially since things can get dinged up during moves, you want to be able to do your final walk-through *after* the seller has moved out.

Things to Know for Your Next Home Purchase

Once you are the proud owner of your first Hippocratic house, having done no harm to your finances during the process, there are some things to know about buying your next home and how your financing and the capital gains taxes can work the second time around.

When You Sell Your Primary Residence, You Don't Have to Reinvest the Profit

Many people don't realize that you don't have to reinvest the cash you obtain from a house sale into your next house, if that house was your primary residence. Let's say you bought your first house for $200,000 and you've got $50,000 equity in it. If you sell that house and get your $50,000 out, you don't have to reinvest that. You can take that and pay off debt with it, and then buy your next house with another physician loan with zero down. In most cases, you won't pay capital gains tax on that money. As long as you've owned the house 24 out of the last 60 months that you've lived in it, there's no capital gains tax and you do not have to reinvest it in your next house.

Your Next House: Can You Still Finance 100%?

There's a "gotcha" with buying a second house using a physician loan. Many lenders don't want to offer 100% financing on a new house and let you keep your old house. If you're already a landlord and you know you are planning to make your previous house a rental property, that's different. The rent from that property will pay the mortgage. But if you want to move out of one house, buy the next one, and then sell the first one later, many lenders frown on that because they're already making a risky loan with no money down. Any loan is a lot riskier when you have two house payments, even if you can afford it. If you're an absentee landlord or an absentee seller, typically the lender will want that house under contract or sold before you buy a new house.

Most lenders will be hesitant to finance the new house at 100% and let you keep your old house. You need to sell it at the same time, either simultaneously with the second purchase or beforehand.

Grand Rounds by Dr. Tammy

Buying your home is just the first expense. You'll need to budget for things like new furniture, minor or major repairs, remodeling, and landscaping. With our newest home, we bought a house that had been on the market for several years and were able to purchase it below market value. We then remodeled it to our taste.

Since we had sold our last house, we had to live in an apartment for six months. Most doctor loans don't allow you to roll in remodeling costs, so make sure you can afford to make it the way you want if you decide to do something like this.

After we moved in, we were surprised with an air conditioner that didn't cool the house, and our washing machine nosedived onto the floor because it wasn't installed properly. Some expenses are anticipated, and others are unexpected. But at the end of the day, we were madly in love with our new house and had an emergency fund to cover these expenses.

Chapter 10 Takeaways

 Moving into your new house takes a little planning. Make sure the lights will be on when you get there by coordinating dates with the seller and setting up utility billing in advance.

 Knowing the right questions to ask can help you avoid many mistakes and wasted money.

 Watch out for common mistakes and avoid them. You can do it right the first time with the right knowledge.

 Check the Resources page at the back of this book for ways you can benefit from the knowledge and experience of others.

CONCLUSION: A MAJOR DECISION DESERVES CAREFUL CONSIDERATION

You probably already realize how much time, effort, planning, and decision-making goes into buying a house. Homeownership is about more than a financial investment. It's also about creating stability, putting down roots, and building a life.

Before you venture down the road of homeownership, ask yourself a few tough questions. Make sure you are up for the challenge of the commitment to owning your house. Your to-do list could grow a mile long once you purchase a house. Even brand-new houses take a lot of work with maintenance and furnishings.

Be realistic about committing your time as well as your resources to a house. If you can barely cover your minimum payments for credit cards and student loans, think twice before taking on homeownership. Buying a house before you clean up your finances is a recipe for disaster.

Do your research, shop around, and compare all your options. You'll rest easier knowing you made the best decision you could, and you may save yourself thousands of dollars in the process.

Grand Rounds by Dr. Tammy

Buying a home for the first or tenth time can be exciting and fun. If you have the right team supporting you, it should be a relatively stress-free experience. Your team can help you with all of these:

 Determine the market price that best fits your budget

 Figure out which type of loan gets you the best interest rate and terms

 Preapprove you as a borrower so you can start looking immediately and make an offer when you find the house of your dreams

 Help you find the house that meets your needs/wants list

As a physician, you have access to loans that many people do not, which can help with wealth-building and financial planning. Your business is very desirable in the real estate industry, so you should surround yourself with a team of people who work to meet your needs. Do not settle for lenders or real estate agents who aren't going out of their way to make your homebuying experience easy and satisfying. Be sure to find people who give you sage advice and counsel. Avoid those who try to upsell you to make a bigger commission. Your home is a main tool for building wealth and financial security.

TERMS

Adjustable-Rate Mortgage (ARM): An adjustable-rate mortgage features a fixed rate for a set period of time (seven or 10 years, for instance). After that time, the interest rate can vary, within limits and time periods, over the remaining course of the loan.

Appraiser: A person who is trained and educated in the methods of determining the value of property, which they perform for a fee. Part of their service is creating an appraisal report containing an opinion as to the value of a property and the reasons behind this opinion.

Closing: The time at which the property is formally sold and transferred from the seller to the buyer. It is at this time that the borrower takes on the loan obligation, pays all closing costs, and receives the title from the seller. Also called the settlement.

Closing Disclosure: A statement that itemizes the services provided to the buyer and the fees charged for those services. This form will be filled out by the person who will conduct the settlement (closing). The buyer can request to see the settlement statement or closing disclosure at least one day prior to the settlement date. Also known as a HUD-1 settlement statement.

Comparative Market Analysis (CMA): In real estate, the practice of comparing price, size, number of beds and baths, lot size, and other amenities for recently sold properties to assist in determining the current market value for a house. Also known as "comps."

Credit Report Fee: This fee covers the cost of a credit report that shows your credit history. The lender uses the information in a credit report to assess someone's credit worthiness.

Debt-to-Income Ratio (DTI): The ratio of how much debt you have compared to the amount of income you earn. This is important for physicians to know because the lender often does not include student loan payments in their calculations for how much they are willing to loan you.

Default: The inability to pay monthly mortgage payments in a timely manner or to otherwise meet the mortgage terms.

Delinquency: A status resulting from failure of a borrower to make timely mortgage payments under a loan agreement.

Down Payment: The portion of a house's purchase price paid in cash, as a certified check or wired funds, and that is not part of the mortgage loan.

Earnest Money Deposit: Money put down (often into an escrow account) to show that the prospective buyer is serious about purchasing the house. It often becomes part of the down payment if the offer is accepted. If the offer is rejected, the earnest money deposit will be returned, or it may be forfeited if the buyer does not follow through with the contracted deal.

Escrow Account: An impound account usually set up by the lender or loan servicer for holding a portion of the monthly mortgage payment that is deposited to cover annual charges for homeowners insurance, mortgage insurance (if applicable), and property taxes. Escrow accounts are also set up to hold earnest money deposits until the closing, and these may be set up by the title company.

Escrow Agent: A person or entity holding documents and funds in a transfer of real property, acting for both parties pursuant to instructions. Typically the agent is a person (often an attorney), escrow company, or title company, depending on local practices which vary by state.

Fannie Mae: Fannie Mae (the Federal National Mortgage Association, FNMA) and Freddie Mac (Federal Home Loan Mortgage Corporation, FHLMC) are government-sponsored enterprises (GSE) created by the U.S. Congress to make home mortgages more accessible to people with moderate income. These entities guarantee conventional mortgage loans and also buy them and repackage them as mortgage-backed securities (MBS), which are purchased by institutions such as insurance companies, pension funds, and investment banks. This practice returns the borrowed funds to mortgage lenders, allowing lenders to create more loans. Secondary market loans, which are the majority of conventional mortgage loans, are what make up mortgage-backed securities.

You can read more about the history of Fannie Mae and Freddie Mac at https://www.investopedia.com/articles/investing/091814/fannie-mae-what-it-does-and-how-it-operates.asp

FHA (Federal Housing Administration): A federal agency that insures mortgage loans and sets standards for construction and underwriting.

Flood Certification Fee: A fee for assessing whether a property is located in a flood-prone area.

Foreclosure: A legal process involving the sale of a mortgaged property to pay the loan of the defaulting borrower.

Government Recording and Transfer Charge: Fees for legally recording the deed and mortgage for a purchased property. These fees may be paid by the buyer or by the seller, depending upon the terms of the sales agreement.

Homeowners Insurance or Home Hazard Insurance: An insurance policy for protecting a house and the owner's possessions inside from serious loss such as theft or fire. This insurance is typically required by all lenders to protect their investment and must be obtained before closing on the mortgage loan.

House Inspection: An inspection of the mechanical, electrical, and structural aspects of a house. The buyer will pay a fee for this inspection, and the inspector will provide the buyer with a written report evaluating the condition of the house.

Interest: The fee charged by the lender for the use of the lender's money.

Interest Rate: The charge by the lender for borrowing money, expressed as a percentage.

Itemized Fee Sheet: An estimate of the settlement charges that will be incurred at closing; it also contains other information about the loan. An itemized fee sheet is simply a condensed version of a loan estimate and the fees shown are not guaranteed. This can be useful to request when shopping with lenders, and you can assume the fees are reasonable estimates. You don't want to go through a complete application to see what their fees look like, so you ask for the fee sheet instead. Also called a good faith estimate (GFE).

Lender Inspection Fees: This charge covers inspections, often of newly constructed housing, made by employees of the lender or by an outside inspector.

Lien: A public record that states a charge has been placed upon or against your property, such as a house, to satisfy a debt legally owed to someone.

Loan Estimate: A complete listing of all closing costs and related fees you will be paying at settlement (closing). The loan estimate will have the same numbers as the fee sheet, however the fee sheet is not guaranteed and the lender is committed to the numbers in the loan estimate—they have to close based on those numbers.

Loan-to-Value Ratio (LTV): A percentage calculated by dividing the amount to be borrowed by the price or appraised value of the house to be purchased, whichever is less. The loan-to-value ratio is used to qualify borrowers for a mortgage, and the higher the LTV, the tighter the qualification guidelines will be for certain mortgage programs. You can reduce the LTV ratio by paying a bigger down payment—no down payment equals 100% LTV. Low loan-to-value ratios are considered below 80% and loans for these will carry lower interest rates since borrowers are considered lower risk. A 20% down payment gives you an 80% LTV.

Mortgage: The transfer of an interest (ownership) in property to a lender as a security for a debt. This interest may be transferred with a *deed of trust* in some states. It is also a lien against a property (as for securing a loan) that becomes void upon full payment or performance according to stipulated terms.

Mortgage Insurance Premium (MIP): Specific to FHA loans, the private mortgage insurance (PMI) that is required to meet the guidelines of an FHA loan.

Origination Fee: A fee charged to the borrower by the loan originator for making a mortgage loan.

Origination Services: Any service involved in the creation of a mortgage loan, including but not limited to the taking of the loan application, loan processing, and the underwriting and funding of the loan. Also includes the processing and administrative services required to perform these functions.

Payment Shock: A scenario in which monthly mortgage payments on an adjustable-rate mortgage (ARM) rise so high that the borrower may not be able to afford the payments.

PITI (Principal, Interest, Taxes, and Insurance): The four elements of a monthly mortgage payment; payments of principal and interest go directly toward repaying the loan or the interest fees on the loan, while the portion that covers taxes and insurance goes into an escrow account to cover the fees when they are due.

Pest Inspection: An inspection for termites or other pest infestations of a house. This inspection is frequently required by the lender prior to closing (settlement).

Point(s): Amount of money paid to reduce the interest rate on a loan. A point is usually equal to 1% of the loan amount.

Prepaid Items: Lenders often require the prepayment of items such as insurance premiums for private mortgage insurance (PMI), homeowners insurance, and real estate taxes.

Prepayment Penalty: A fee charged if the mortgage loan is paid (in whole or in part) before the scheduled due date.

Private Mortgage Insurance (PMI): Insurance the buyer pays to benefit the bank that is loaning them money. Not required for all types of mortgage loans, but typically if the buyer contributes less than 20% of the purchase price as a down payment (and therefore has less than 20% equity in the house), the lender will require PMI. PMI is provided by a third-party insurer for the benefit of the bank. The lender may require payment of the first year's PMI premiums or a lump sum premium that covers the life of the loan in advance at settlement (closing).

Recording and Transfer Charges: These charges include fees paid to the local government for filing official records of a real estate transaction.

Sales Agreement: The contract signed by a buyer and the seller stating the terms and conditions under which a property will be sold. It may also be called an "Agreement of Sale" or "Purchase Contract."

Settlement: The time at which the property is formally sold and transferred from the seller to the buyer. It is at this time that the borrower takes on the loan obligation, pays all closing costs, and receives the title from the seller. Also called the closing.

Settlement/Closing Agent: In some states, a settlement agent, or closing agent, handles the real estate transaction when someone buys or sells a house. It may also be an attorney or a title agent. He or she oversees all legal documents, fee payments, and other details of transferring the property to ensure that the conditions of the contract have been met and appropriate real estate taxes have been paid.

Settlement Costs/Closing Costs: The customary costs above and beyond the sales price of the property that must be paid to cover the transfer of ownership at closing; these costs generally vary by geographic location and are typically detailed to the borrower at the time the itemized fee sheet (or good faith estimate, GFE) is given.

Survey Fee: A fee for obtaining a drawing of the property to be purchased, showing the location of the lot, any structures, and any encroachments. The survey fee is usually paid by the borrower (buyer).

Tax Certificate: Official proof of payment of taxes due provided at the time of transfer of property title by the state or local government.

Tax Service Fee: This fee covers the cost of the lender engaging a third party to monitor and handle the payment of the property tax bills. This is done to ensure that the tax payments are made on time and to prevent tax liens from occurring.

Title Insurance: Insurance that protects the lender against any title dispute that may arise over the purchased property. Through a title search, the lender verifies who the actual property owners are and whether the property is free of liens. The title search company then issues title insurance, which protects the title of the property against any unpaid mortgages and judgments. In case a claim is made against the property, the title insurance provides legal protection and pays for court fees and related costs. The buyer may also purchase owner's title insurance, which protects the homeowner.

Title Service Fees: Title service fees include charges for title search and title insurance if required. This fee also includes the services of a title or settlement agent.

Tolerance Category: The maximum amount by which the charges for a category or categories of settlement cost may exceed the amount of the estimate for such category or categories on the itemized fee sheet (good faith estimate, GFE). When the originator selects and identifies the provider of services, these charges may only increase 10% in the aggregate. If the borrower selects a provider that is not on the written list provided by the loan originator, the lender is not subject to any tolerance restrictions for that service.

VA (Veterans Administration): The United States government's department of Veterans Administration.

RESOURCES

1. For more information on all aspects of physician finances and to reach Doug Crouse for advice, visit DougCrouse.com or call or text at 816-728-3631.

2. *Financial Residency* podcast: http://www.financialresidency.com/itunes

3. Rent-to-buy calculator: https://www.nytimes.com/interactive /2014/upshot/buy-rent-calculator.html

4. Student loan repayment options: see the free tool at www.financialresidency.com/loanbuddy

5. Free credit reports as recommended by the FTC (Federal Trade Commission) can be obtained from all three reporting agencies once every 12 months from https://www.annualcreditreport.com/index.action

6. More on how to get your credit score: https://www.consumerfinance.gov/ask-cfpb/i-got-my-free-credit-reports-but-they-do-not-include-my-credit-scores-can-i-get-my-credit-score-for-free-too-en-6/

7. Mortgage calculator: https://www.mortgagecalculator.org or https://www.mortgagecalculator.org/calculators/mortgage-payment-calculator.php or https://www.bankrate.com/calculators/mortgages/amortization-calculator.aspx

8. For more information on VA loans: https://www.va.gov/housing-assistance/home-loans/eligibility/

9.   Information on VA home loan limits: https://www.va.gov/
      housing-assistance/home-loans/loan-limits/

10.   For more information on income limits and geographic regions for
      USDA loans: https://www.rd.usda.gov/files/RD-DirectLimitMap.pdf

11.   For examples of loan estimate and closing disclosure forms, visit
      DougCrouse.com

ACKNOWLEDGMENTS

I would like to thank my wife and co-author, Tammy Crouse, and of course Ryan Inman for all their great input in helping me put this book together.

I'd also like to thank the team at Aloha Publishing, including Maryanna Young, Megan Terry, Jennifer Regner, Heather Goetter, Beth Berger, and Terina Treloar.

ABOUT THE AUTHORS

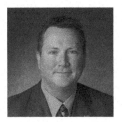 **Doug Crouse** is an experienced mortgage loan originator who loves helping his clients with their house financing needs. He has lived in Kansas City since 1990 and began his mortgage career in 1999. Doug has helped thousands of borrowers over the years find the houses of their dreams.

He specializes in physician loans and has closed on more than $194M in residential properties in one year. He and his physician wife, Tammy, have bought three homes together.

Doug also had a real estate broker license, earlier in his career, and focused on selling houses at that time. He has closed approximately 125.

When he's not helping clients, he enjoys going to KC Chiefs games. He and his son have had season tickets since 2001.

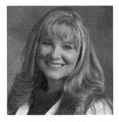 **Dr. Tammy Crouse** is a hospitalist specializing in family medicine. She received her medical degree from Kansas City University College of Osteopathic Medicine and is affiliated with multiple hospitals in Missouri. She has been in practice more than 15 years.

Doug and Tammy enjoy traveling to anywhere with a beach. Their children are grown and they have two adorable Chihuahua mix rescue dogs that rule the Crouse house.

CONNECT WITH ME

If you are a physician or other healthcare professional and are thinking about buying a house, I would love to help you get into the house that will make you happy. I work in multiple states and can recommend great professionals to you in other states. Reach out to me by visiting DougCrouse.com or FinancialResidency.com to access all the financial and homebuying resources that are available to you.

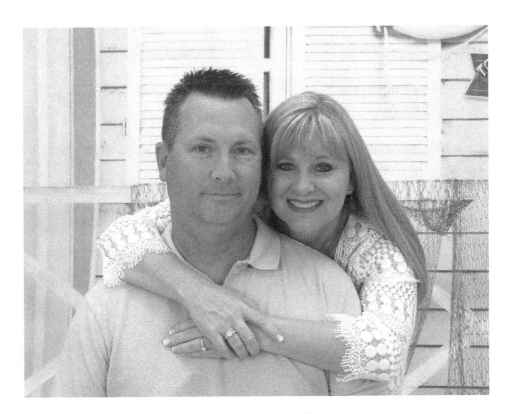

Financial Residency podcast

FinancialResidency.com/podcast

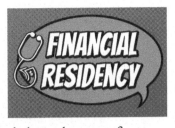

You spent decades in school to get to where you are as a doctor, but during medical school and residency, you probably didn't receive an education dedicated to your finances. Don't worry, that's where the podcast comes in. Think of it as your financial residency without the long hours and sleepless nights. You'll understand how you make money, how you spend money, how your hard-earned money can work for you, and how to protect yourself and your family. It's okay to not know the difference between a Roth IRA and a 403(b) or know which 529 plan is best. I will simplify highly complex concepts and translate industry jargon into plain English. Are you ready to take action and make smarter, more informed financial decisions? Great—let's do this! Let your financial residency begin. Find us on all the major podcast players: Apple, Stitcher, iHeart Radio, Spotify, Google, and more!

Physician Wealth Services

PhysicianWealthServices.com

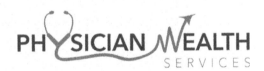

Physician Wealth Services (PWS) is a fee-only financial planning practice helping physician families take control of their finances to position themselves for a bright financial future. We help physicians sleep well at night knowing they have a trusted advisor who is guiding them toward financial independence. Our goal is to take care of you while you take care of your patients. We are accessible when you are—in the evenings after you get your kids to bed, during your commute home, or between patients. Short of the overnight shift, consider us on call. Most importantly, we are fiduciaries for our clients and we work exclusively with physicians all around the country.

For more information, go to PhysicianWealthServices.com
FB Group: www.facebook.com/groups/physicianfinance
Twitter: @physicianwealth
Instagram: www.instagram.com/financialresidency

Check out this book from Financial Residency...

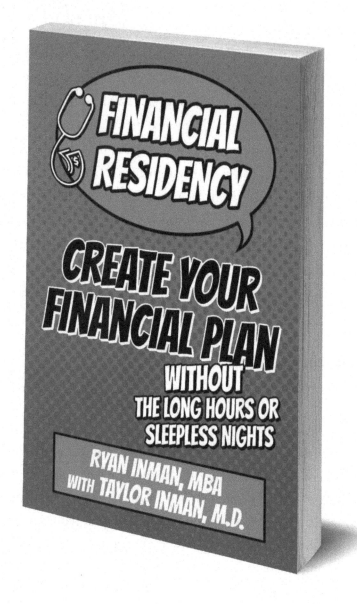

Available on Amazon.com and other great online retailers,
FinancialResidency.com, and AlohaPublishing.com